PALEO DIET FOR

2 Books in 1: 200+ High-protein and Low-carb Recipes to Discover the Secrets of Rapid Weight Loss and A Healthy Lifestyle Using the Paleo Diet!

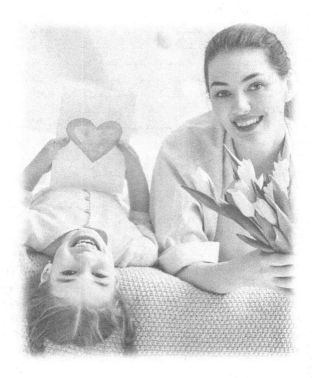

By

Robert Baker

TABLE OF CONTENT

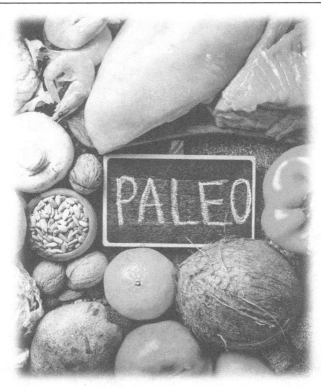

It's an epidemic in this country: people are overweight, tired, and eating poorly. The American diet is full of carbs, sugars, and processed foods that make us fat, feel malnourished, and too tired to do anything with our lives.

If you picked up this book, you're looking for a change. She's looking for a way to eat healthier and feel better. She also wants to lose weight. She realizes that the current Western diet is not working for her. Well, this book has the answer she's looking for.

Eat like a cave dweller! People refer to the paleo diet as the caveman diet because it is based on how humans ate over 10,000 years ago, before the advent of agriculture. People ate what was available through hunting and foraging, namely meat, fruits, vegetables, and nuts. Dairy products, carbohydrates, and anything else that was processed was not available to them.

Eating like a cave dweller has many benefits, the biggest of which is that they will be healthier and lose weight. It may take some dedication to give up the foods he is used to, but the results are more than worth it. Imagine being at a healthy weight for your body, having the energy to do all the activities you dream of, and feeling lean and mean, like the caveman of old.

He can lose weight. He can eat healthily. He can take control of his life. By eating the paleo diet, he will have all of these things.

THE BENEFITS OF THE PALEO DIET FOR WOMEN

The paleo diet plan is a dietary program that mimics the way prehistoric people could eat. It involves the consumption of whole foods that people could scavenge or gather.

Paleo diet plan promoters reject new diet programs that are usually full of processed foods. They think that the time of how hunter-gatherers consumed might cause fewer health problems.

The paleo diet plan is not safe for everyone. Doctors have no idea about its results on children, pregnant women, or older adults. Individuals with persistent problems, such as inflammatory bowel disease, should talk to a doctor before trying a paleo diet plan. This manual explores paleo principles and a 7-day paleo diet meal to follow. Read on to understand how to consume like our ancestors. The paleo diet plan focuses on consuming foods that may have been obtainable as early as the Paleolithic era.

Additionally, the paleo diet plan is called the rock age diet plan, hunter-gatherer diet plan, or caveman diet plan. Before contemporary agriculture developed about 10,000 years ago, people usually ate foods they could hunt or gather, such as fish, liver organs, fruits, vegetables, peanuts, and seeds. The introduction of modern agriculture changed the way people ate. Dairy products, dry beans, and grains became a part of people's food plans.

Proponents of the paleo diet plan believe that the body did not evolve to process dairy, dry beans, and grains. Consuming these foods could increase the threat of specific health problems, such as cardiovascular disease, overweight, and diabetes.

Health advantages of paleo

Individuals state that the paleo eating plan offers numerous health advantages, such as promoting weight reduction, reducing the possibility of diabetes, and decreasing blood pressure. In this area, we review the scientific evidence to find out what studies facilitate these claims:

Excess weight loss

A 2008 research study found that 14 healthy volunteers achieved an average weight reduction of 2.3 pounds by following a paleo diet plan for three weeks.

In 2009, researchers compared the consequences of the paleo diet plan with the diabetes diet plan on 13 people with type 2 diabetes. A little research discovered that consuming the paleo method decreased the individuals' body weight and waist area. The 2014 research on 70 post-menopausal women with weight problems found that executing a paleo diet plan helped individual lose weight after six months.

However, right after 24 months, there was simply no difference in weight reduction between individuals following a paleo diet and those following regular Nordic nutritional suggestions. These findings state that some other healthy diet programs could be just as effective in advertising weight reduction.

The authors of the 2017 review noted that this paleo diet plan helped reduce weight for a while, but they understood that this result was due to calorie restriction or eating fewer calories. Overall, the study shows that the paleo diet plan can help people lose weight initially, but that other diet plans that reduce calorie consumption could be effective. Also, the study is essential before doctors recommend the paleo diet plan for weight reduction. Currently, doctors recommend following exercise and a calorie-controlled diet even more to lose excess weight.

Decrease the risk of diabetes

Does running a paleo diet program reduce the danger of getting diabetes? The results of some preliminary research are usually encouraging. The level of insulin resistance is a dangerous element of diabetes. Improving one's level of insulin sensitivity reduces the likelihood of leading to diabetes and helps those with diabetes decrease signs and symptoms. A 2015 study compared the consequences of the paleo diet plan with those of a diet plan based on the American Diabetes Association's recommendations on people who have type 2 diabetes. While both diet plans improved individuals' metabolic health, the paleo diet plan improved insulin resistance and control of blood sugar levels. A 2009 study of nine sedentary volunteers without obesity found that the paleo diet plan improved insulin awareness.

There is a need for a more recent study on the paleo diet plan and diabetes. However, the evidence so far shows that eating just like a hunter-gatherer can improve insulin sensitivity.

Decrease blood pressure

Increased blood pressure is a factor that leads to the onset of cardiovascular disease. Many believe that the paleo eating plan can help keep blood pressure balanced and increase coronary artery wellness.

A 2010 research on 14 healthy volunteers found that following a paleo eating plan for three weeks improved systolic blood pressure. It additionally reduced excess weight and body mass catalog (BMI). The analysis does not add a group of handles, and yet the results are usually not conclusive. A 2017 research reported results similar to the first ones obtained. Researchers compared the consequences of the paleo diet plan with those of a diet plan that Dutch well-being authorities recommend on 48 individuals with characteristics of metabolic symptoms, a disorder that increases the danger of cardiovascular disease.

The results showed how the paleo diet plan reduced blood pressure and liver lipid levels, both of which can improve body wellness.

Although preliminary studies state that the paleo diet can reduce blood pressure and support heart health, more recent supporting studies will be essential to conclude.

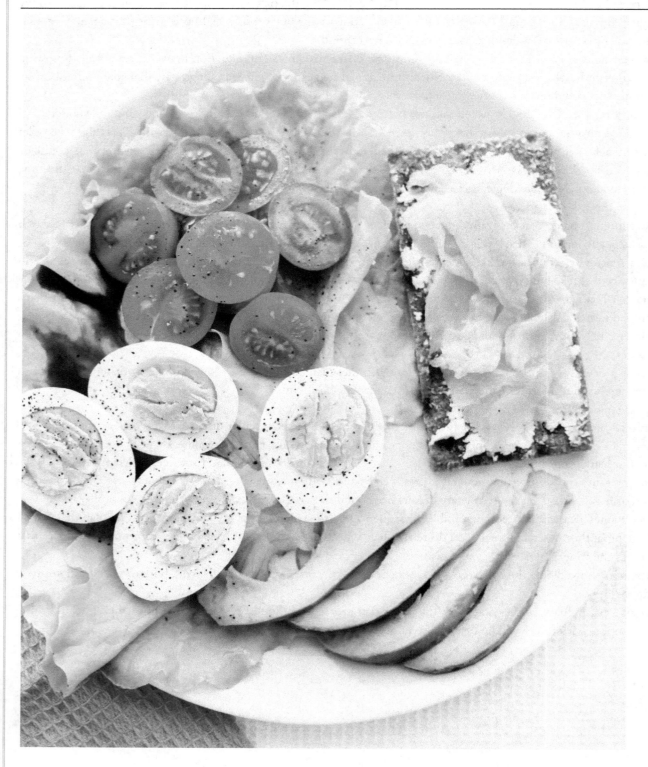

1) Easy Salmon Sheet Pan Dinner

Preparation Time: 30 minutes

Servings: 4

Ingredients:

- ✓ 1 1/2 cups cherry tomatoes
- ✓ 1 large fennel bulb, sliced lengthwise into steaks
- ✓ 1 zucchini, cut into coins

Ingredients:

- ✓ olive oil
- ✓ 2 lemons, halved
- ✓ 1 1/2 pounds salmon filet, whole or cut into filets
- ✓ kosher salt, to taste

Directions:

- ❖ Preheat oven to 450 degrees F.
- ❖ Place the first 5 ingredients on a sheet pan and toss with olive oil to coat and salt to taste.
- ❖ Distribute the vegetables around the pan in a single layer and bake for 10 minutes.
- ❖ Remove the sheet pan from the oven and push some of the vegetables to the side to make space for the salmon fillets.

- ❖ Season the salmon with salt and bake for 12-15 additional minutes (depending on the thickness of your salmon fillets).
- ❖ Turn the broiler on for 2 minutes or until the vegetables are golden.
- ❖ Place salmon and vegetables on a plate and offer a lemon half for squeezing over fish and vegetables.

2) Delicious Turkey Zucchini Burgers with Yogurt-Sumac Sauce

Preparation Time: 20 minutes

Servings: 4

Ingredients:

- ✓ For the burgers:
- ✓ 1 pound ground turkey, light or dark meat
- ✓ 1 large zucchini, coarsely grated
- ✓ 3 scallions, thinly sliced
- ✓ 1 large egg
- ✓ 2 tbsps chopped mint
- ✓ 2 tbsp chopped cilantro
- ✓ 2 garlic cloves, minced
- ✓ 1 tsp ground cumin

Ingredients:

- ✓ 1 teaspoon kosher salt
- ✓ olive oil, for greasing the pan
- ✓ 8 mini hamburger buns
- ✓ For the yogurt sauce:
- ✓ 1 cup greek yogurt
- ✓ 1 teaspoon grated lemon zest
- ✓ 1 tbsp lemon juice
- ✓ 1 garlic clove, minced
- ✓ 1 tbsp olive oil
- ✓ 2 teaspoons sumac
- ✓ 1/2 teaspoon kosher salt

Directions:

- ❖ In a large bowl combine first 9 ingredients.
- ❖ Mix well.
- ❖ With dampened hands form the mixture into burgers about 1 inch thick. You can do small slider size or regular size burgers.

- ❖ In a large saute pan or stove top grill over medium, add 1-2 tbsps olive oil and add the burger patties.
- ❖ Cook burgers 3-4 minutes on each side for small slider burgers or 5-6 minutes on each side for larger burgers.
- ❖ Place all the sauce ingredients in a small bowl and stir to combine.
- ❖ Place the burgers on buns and top with the yogurt-sumac sauce.

3) Special Hearty Breakfast

Preparation Time: 35 minutes

Servings: 2

Ingredients:

- ✓ 3 lb. pork roast, boneless
- ✓ 2 tsp. cumin, ground
- ✓ 1 tsp. red pepper flakes, crushed
- ✓ A pinch of sea salt and black pepper
- ✓ 1 tsp. oregano, dried
- ✓ Juice from 1 orange
- ✓ Orange peel from 1 orange, grated

Directions:

- ❖ Put roast in your instant pot.
- ❖ Add cumin, pepper flakes, salt, pepper, oregano, orange juice, orange peel, garlic, yellow onion, bay leaf and oil and rub roast well.
- ❖ Cover instant pot and cook on high for 20 minutes.

Ingredients:

- ✓ 6 garlic cloves, minced
- ✓ 1 yellow onion, chopped
- ✓ 1 bay leaf
- ✓ 1 tbsp. avocado oil
- ✓ 2 tsp. cilantro, chopped
- ✓ 1 butter lettuce head, torn
- ✓ 2 radishes, sliced
- ✓ 2 avocados, pitted, peeled and sliced
- ✓ 1 cup Paleo salsa
- ✓ 2 jalapeños, chopped
- ✓ 3 limes, quartered
- ❖ Transfer roast to a cutting board, leave aside to cool down a bit, shred and divide among plates.
- ❖ Also divide lettuce leaves, radishes, avocado slices, jalapeños and lime wedges.
- ❖ Sprinkle cilantro, divide salsa on top and serve for breakfast.

Nutrition: Calories275 | Fat: 4g | Carbs: 5g | Protein: 14g | Fiber: 3g | Sugar: 0g

4) **Easy Breakfast Quiche**

Preparation Time: 30 minutes   **Servings: 2**

Ingredients:

- ✓ 1 cup water
- ✓ 6 eggs, whisked
- ✓ A pinch of black pepper
- ✓ ½ cup coconut milk

Directions:

- ❖ Put the water in your instant pot and add the steamer basket inside.
- ❖ Put bacon, sausage and ham in a bowl, mix and spread on the bottom of a quiche dish.

Ingredients:

- ✓ 4 bacon slices, cooked and crumbled
- ✓ 1 cup sausage, cooked and ground
- ✓ ½ cup ham, chopped
- ✓ 2 green onions, chopped
- ❖ In a bowl, mix eggs with black pepper, coconut milk and green onions and whisk well.
- ❖ Pour this over meat, spread, place inside the pot, cover and cook on high for 30 minutes
- ❖ Slice, divide among plates and serve.

Nutrition: Calories243 | Fat: 3g | Carbs: 6g | Protein: 12g | Fiber: 1g | Sugar: 0g

5) Wonderful Omelette

Preparation Time: 18 minutes

Servings: 2

Ingredients:

- ✓ 4 oz. sweet potatoes, cut into medium fries
- ✓ 6 eggs
- ✓ A pinch of sea salt and black pepper
- ✓ 1 tbsp. olive oil
- ✓ ¼ cup scallions, chopped

Ingredients:

- ✓ 1 garlic clove, minced
- ✓ ¼ cup coconut milk
- ✓ 1 tsp. Paleo tomato paste
- ✓ 1 and ½ cups water
- ✓ 1 green bell pepper, chopped
- ❖ Pour this over eggs mix, stir well and spread everything on top of sweet potato fries.
- ❖ Put the water in your instant pot, add the steamer basket inside and place the eggs mix in the basket.
- ❖ Cover, cook on high for 18 minutes, slice, divide among plates and serve hot.

Directions:

- ❖ Grease a heat proof dish with the oil and spread sweet potato fries on the bottom.
- ❖ In a bowl, mix eggs with salt, pepper, scallions, garlic and bell pepper and whisk well.
- ❖ In another bowl, mix coconut milk with tomato paste and stir.

Nutrition: Calories153 | Fat: 7g | Carbs: 5g | Protein: 15g | Fiber: 2g | Sugar: 0g

6) Special Pumpkin and Apple Butter

Preparation Time: 10 minutes

Servings: 2

Ingredients:

- ✓ 3 apples, peeled, cored and chopped
- ✓ 30 oz. pumpkin puree
- ✓ 1 tbsp. pumpkin pie spice

Ingredients:

- ✓ 1 cup honey
- ✓ 12 oz. apple cider

- ❖ Divide into jars, seal them and serve for breakfast when ever you want.

Directions:

- ❖ Put pumpkin puree in your instant pot.
- ❖ Add apples, pumpkin pie spice, cider and honey, stir well, cover and cook on high for 10 minutes

Nutrition: Calories100 | Fat: 3g | Carbs: 4g | Protein: 6g | Fiber: 1g | Sugar: 0g

7) Easy Breakfast Spinach Delight

Preparation Time: 30 minutes

Servings: 2

Ingredients:

- ✓ 1 lb. mustard leaves
- ✓ 1 lb. spinach, torn
- ✓ 2 tbsp. olive oil
- ✓ A small ginger piece, grated
- ✓ 2 yellow onions, chopped
- ✓ 4 garlic cloves, minced
- ✓ 1 tsp. cumin, ground

Ingredients:

- ✓ 1 tsp. coriander, ground
- ✓ 1 tsp. garam masala
- ✓ A pinch of cayenne pepper
- ✓ ½ tsp. turmeric
- ✓ A pinch of black pepper
- ✓ A pinch of fenugreek leaves, dried

- ❖ Add spinach and mustard leaves, stir gently, cover and cook on high for 15 minutes.
- ❖ Divide into bowls and serve for breakfast.

Directions:

- ❖ Set your instant pot on sauté mode, add oil and heat it up.
- ❖ Add onion, garlic, ginger, coriander, cumin, garam masala, turmeric, cayenne pepper, black pepper and fenugreek, stir and cook for 5 minutes.

Nutrition: Calories200 | Fat: 3g | Carbs: 5g | Protein: 7g | Fiber: 2g | Sugar: 0g

8) Special and Amazing Bacon and Sweet Potato Breakfast

Preparation Time: 10 minutes

Servings: 2

Ingredients:

- ✓ 2 lbs. sweet potatoes, cubed
- ✓ A pinch of salt and black pepper
- ✓ 3 bacon strips

Ingredients:

- ✓ 2 tbsp. water
- ✓ 2 tsp. parsley, dried
- ✓ 1 tsp. garlic powder
- ✓ 4 eggs, fried for serving
- ❖ Divide among plates next to fried eggs and serve.

Directions:

- ❖ In your instant pot, mix sweet potatoes with bacon, salt, pepper, water, parsley and garlic powder, stir, cover and cook on high for 10 minutes.

Nutrition: Calories 200 | Fat: 2g | Carbs: 6g | Protein: 8g | Fiber: 2g | Sugar: 0g

9) Easy and Spiced Carrot Cauliflower Soup

Preparation Time: 40 minutes

Servings: 6-8

Ingredients:

- ✓ 1 tbsp olive oil
- ✓ 1 small onion, chopped
- ✓ 5 cups warm water
- ✓ 2 tbsp vegetable bouillon*
- ✓ 1 head cauliflower, chopped (about 4 cups)

Ingredients:

- ✓ 3 cups peeled and chopped carrots (about 8 medium carrots)
- ✓ 1 1/2 tsp curry powder
- ✓ 1 teaspoon ground cinnamon
- ✓ 1 teaspoon garam masala
- ✓ 1 teaspoon kosher salt
- ❖ Bring to a boil, cover, and reduce heat to simmer for 15-20 minutes, or until the vegetables are fork tender.
- ❖ Using an immersion blender or standing blender, puree all of the ingredients until smooth.

Directions:

- ❖ Heat the oil in a large saucepan over medium heat and cook the onions for 3 minutes, or until soft.
- ❖ Dissolve the vegetable bouillon in the water and add to the pot.
- ❖ Add the remaining ingredients to the pot and stir to combine.

Preparation Time: 25 minutes

Ingredients:

- ✓ dressing:
- ✓ 1/4 cup plain unsweetened almond milk
- ✓ 1/2 cup paleo mayo homemade or store bought
- ✓ 1 Tbsps lemon juice
- ✓ 1 tsp fresh minced dill or 1/4 tsp dried
- ✓ 1 garlic clove minced
- ✓ 2 Tbsp chopped chives
- ✓ Sea Salt and black pepper to taste
- ✓ Salmon
- ✓ 3/4 tsp sea salt
- ✓ 1/8 tsp black pepper

Ingredients:

- ✓ 1 lb individual salmon fillets skin on or off (3-4 fillets)
- ✓ 3/4 tsp garlic powder
- ✓ 3/4 tsp onion powder
- ✓ 3/4 tsp smoked paprika
- ✓ 1 Tbsp bacon fat avocado oil, or ghee
- ✓ salad:
- ✓ 6 cups mixed greens of choice roughly chopped
- ✓ 1 cup cherry tomatoes halved
- ✓ 6 Slices bacon cooked until crisp and crumbled or chopped
- ✓ 1 medium avocado thinly sliced
- ✓ 1 small red onion thinly sliced
- ❖ Add oil to the skillet. In a skillet, place the salmon skin side down (if you chose skin) and cook about 3 minutes on each side, adjusting for preference and thickness.
- ❖ If grilling, brush grill with oil and place the salmon flesh side down on the hot grill.
- ❖ Cook about 3 minutes, then carefully flip and cook skin side down for another 3-4 minutes, adjusting for thickness and preference.
- ❖ Remove to a plate and assemble the salad.
- ❖ Layer the greens with tomatoes, bacon, sliced avocado and red onion and place salmon on top.
- ❖ Drizzle all over with as much of the dressing as you like and garnish with extra chives if desired. Serve right away. Enjoy!

Directions:

- ❖ dressing:
- ❖ Whisk together the almond milk, mayo, lemon juice and dill until smooth.
- ❖ Stir in the garlic and chives, then season to taste with sea salt and black pepper.
- ❖ salmon:
- ❖ Pat the fillets dry with paper towel. In a small bowl, mix together all the seasonings. You can make the salmon on the stovetop in a skillet or on the grill. If grilling, brush generously all over with the oil before beginning. If pan frying, the oil is for the skillet.
- ❖ Heat the grill or skillet to medium high heat.

11) Easy Garlic Butter Steak Bites

Preparation Time: 20 minutes

Servings: 2-4

Ingredients:

- ✓ ½ tbsp avocado oil
- ✓ 2 pounds of steak, cut into small bite size pieces
- ✓ 2 teaspoons salt
- ✓ ½ teaspoon freshly ground black pepper

Directions:

- ❖ Season the steak bites with salt, pepper, and red pepper flakes and stir until well coated.
- ❖ Heat a large skillet over medium-high heat.
- ❖ Add the avocado oil to the hot skillet and then add the steak in a single layer.
- ❖ Cook the steak bites for 3-4 minutes until brown, stirring occasionally. You may have to do this in batches depending on the size of your skillet.

Ingredients:

- ✓ ½ teaspoon red pepper flakes (optional)
- ✓ 2 tbsps butter or ghee
- ✓ 6 cloves minced garlic
- ✓ ¼ cup chopped parsley
- ✓ green onion, for garnish
- ❖ Once the steak is brown, remove it from the pan.
- ❖ Remove any excess water from the skillet and then add the butter or ghee to the pan.
- ❖ Next add the garlic and saute for 1 minute.
- ❖ Add the steak back to the pan and cook for 1-2 minutes stirring to coat it in the butter sauce.
- ❖ Remove the pan from the heat and stir in the chopped parsley.
- ❖ Garnish with green onion and serve immediately.

12) Special Shrimp Fried Cauliflower Rice

Preparation Time: 25 minutes

Servings: 2-4

Ingredients:

- ✓ 1 lb medium-large raw shrimp peeled and deveined
- ✓ 1 tsp tapioca flour or arrowroot*
- ✓ Sea salt and black pepper
- ✓ 2 Tbsp avocado oil or ghee divided
- ✓ 3 eggs whisked
- ✓ 1 1/2 cups carrots diced
- ✓ 1 bunch scallions white and green parts separated - thinly sliced

Directions:

- ❖ Have all ingredients prepped and ready to go before beginning.
- ❖ In a bowl, toss the shrimp with the tapioca or arrowroot, salt and pepper. Heat a large nonstick skillet over medium high heat.
- ❖ Once hot, add 1 Tbsp avocado oil or ghee.
- ❖ Add shrimp in a single layer and cook 1-2 minutes per side until opaque, careful not to overcook.
- ❖ Remove to a plate and turn the heat to medium.
- ❖ With the skillet over medium heat, add the whisked eggs and cook until just set, breaking them up with your spatula.
- ❖ Set them aside with the shrimp.
- ❖ Add the second tbsp of oil or ghee to the skillet and adjust heat medium high.

Ingredients:

- ✓ 1 inch chunk fresh ginger peeled and minced about 2 tsp
- ✓ 3 cloves garlic minced
- ✓ 12 oz cauliflower rice fresh or frozen. If frozen, thaw first.
- ✓ 1/4 cup coconut aminos (this is a paleo and Whole30 friendly equivalent of soy sauce)
- ✓ 1 tbsp pure sesame oil
- ✓ Sea salt to taste
- ❖ Add the diced carrots and cook, stirring, 3-4 minutes or until fork tender.
- ❖ Then add in the white part of the scallions, ginger, and garlic and stir to combine.
- ❖ Cook another minute until fragrant.
- ❖ Add in the cauliflower rice, coconut aminos and sesame oil and stir to combine.
- ❖ Cook about 2-3 minutes to soften the cauliflower rice.
- ❖ Add in the shrimp and eggs and stir and cook 30-60 seconds to heat through, then remove from heat.
- ❖ Garnish with the green part of the scallions and additional coconut aminos or salt and pepper to taste.
- ❖ Serve right away. Leftovers can be saved in the sealed container in the refrigerator for up to 4 days. Enjoy

13) Special Thai Chicken Satay

Preparation Time: 30 minutes

Servings: 2-4

Ingredients:

- ✓ Thai chicken satay marinade:
- ✓ 1.5-2 lbs chicken thighs, boneless and skinless
- ✓ 1 tsp turmeric powder
- ✓ 1 tsp coriander powder
- ✓ 0.5 tsp white pepper
- ✓ 0.5 tsp cumin powder

Ingredients:

- ✓ 4 tbsp dairy-free coffee creamer, or melted coconut cream
- ✓ 1 tsp fish sauce
- ✓ 2 tbsp coconut aminos, or 1 tbsp low sodium/gluten-free tamari
- ✓ 2 tsp grated ginger
- ✓ 2 tbsp hot sauce, I use Frank's original hot sauce
- ✓ Avocado oil cooking spray, for the air fryer basket
- ❖ Air fry at 370F (188C) for 15 minutes on the first side and 8-10 minutes the second side or until the chicken is cooked through. Please note that cook time varies, depending on the type of air fryer.

Directions:

- ❖ In a large mixing bowl, marinate the chicken thighs with ingredients from turmeric to hot sauce.
- ❖ Gently mix well and cover the bowl.
- ❖ Store in the fridge for at least 30 minutes or up to 1 day before cooking.
- ❖ To air fry, lightly spray the fryer basket with avocado oil.
- ❖ Slightly drip off the marinade and place the chicken thighs into the basket in one layer with some space between each piece.
- ❖ Please do not over crowd the basket. I cook mine in two batches.

- ❖ To pan fry (stovetop), add 1 tbsp avocado oil to a well-heated skillet.
- ❖ Pan fry 6 minutes the first side and 5-6 minutes the second side over medium heat or until the chicken is cooked through.
- ❖ Serve hot or at room temperature. The chicken is very tender and flavorful and you don't need a dipping sauce however if you like to kick the flavor over the top, try my Paleo Thai "Peanut" sauce.
- ❖ Serve it over a big bowl of salad greens or Keto garlic fried rice!

14) Special Morning Berry-Green Smoothie

Preparation Time: 5 minutes

Servings: 4

Ingredients:

- ✓ 3 cups mixed blueberries and strawberries
- ✓ 1 avocado, pitted and sliced
- ✓ 2 cups unsweetened almond milk

Ingredients:

- ✓ 6 tbsp heavy cream
- ✓ 2 tbsp erythritol
- ✓ 1 cup ice cubes
- ✓ ⅓ cup nuts and seeds mix
- ❖ Blend at high speed until smooth and uniform. Pour the smoothie into drinking glasses and serve immediately.

Directions:

- ❖ Combine the avocado slices, blueberries, strawberries, almond milk, heavy cream, erythritol, ice cubes, nuts, and seeds in a smoothie maker.

Nutrition: Calories Calories 360, Fat 33.3g, Net Carbs 6g, Protein 6g

15) Nut Granola and Smoothie Bowl

Preparation Time: 5 minutes

Servings: 4

Ingredients:
- ✓ 6 cups Greek yogurt
- ✓ 4 tbsp almond butter
- ✓ A handful toasted walnuts

Directions:
- ❖ Combine the Greek yogurt, almond butter, walnuts, cocoa powder, and swerve brown sugar in a smoothie maker. Puree at high speed until smooth and well mixed

Ingredients:
- ✓ 3 tbsp unsweetened cocoa powder
- ✓ 4 tsp swerve brown sugar
- ✓ 2 cups nut granola for topping
- ❖ Share the smoothie into four breakfast bowls, top with a half cup of granola each one, and serve.

Nutrition: Calories 361K, Fat 31.2g, Net Carbs 2g, Protein 13g

16) Morning Almond Shake

Preparation Time: 5 minutes

Servings: 2

Ingredients:
- ✓ 1 ½ cups almond milk
- ✓ 2 tbsp almond butter
- ✓ ½ tsp almond extract
- ✓ ½ tsp cinnamon

Directions:
- ❖ Add almond milk, almond butter, flax meal, almond extract, collagen peptides, a pinch of salt, and stevia to a blender bowl. Blitz until uniform and smooth, about 30 seconds.

Ingredients:
- ✓ 2 tbsp flax meal
- ✓ 1 tbsp collagen peptides
- ✓ A pinch of salt
- ✓ 15 drops of stevia
- ✓ A handful of ice cubes
- ❖ Then taste and adjust flavor as needed, adding more stevia for sweetness or almond butter to the creaminess. Pour in a smoothie glass, add the ice cubes and sprinkle with cinnamon.

Nutrition: Calories Calories 326, Fat: 27g, Net Carbs: 6g, Protein: 19g

17) Delicious Chocolate Protein Coconut Shake

Preparation Time: 5 minutes

Servings: 4

Ingredients:
- ✓ 3 cups flax milk, chilled
- ✓ 3 tsp unsweetened cocoa powder
- ✓ 1 medium avocado, peeled, sliced
- ✓ 1 cup coconut milk, chilled

Directions:
- ❖ Combine the flax milk, cocoa powder, avocado, coconut milk, 3 mint leaves, erythritol, and protein powder into the smoothie maker, and blend for 1 minute to smooth.

Ingredients:
- ✓ 3 mint leaves + extra to garnish
- ✓ 3 tbsp erythritol
- ✓ 1 tbsp low carb protein powder
- ✓ Whipping cream for topping
- ❖ Pour the drink into serving glasses, lightly add some whipping cream on top, and garnish with 1 or 2 mint leaves. Serve immediately.

Nutrition: Calories Calories 265, Fat: 15.5g, Net Carbs: 4g, Protein: 12g

18) Easy Five Greens Smoothie

Preparation Time: 5 minutes

Servings: 4

Ingredients:
- ✓ 6 kale leaves, chopped
- ✓ 3 stalks celery, chopped
- ✓ 1 ripe avocado, skinned and sliced

Directions:
- ❖ In a blender, add the kale, celery, avocado, and ice cubes, and blend for 45 seconds. Add the spinach and cucumber, and process for another 45 seconds until smooth

Ingredients:
- ✓ 2 cups spinach, chopped
- ✓ 1 cucumber, peeled and chopped
- ✓ Chia seeds to garnish
- ❖ Pour the smoothie into glasses, garnish with chia seeds, and serve the drink immediately.

Nutrition: Calories Calories 124, Fat 7.8g, Net Carbs 2.9g, Protein 3.2g

19) Special Dark Chocolate Smoothie

Preparation Time: 10 minutes

Servings: 2

Ingredients:
- ✓ ½ cup pecans
- ✓ ¾ cup coconut milk
- ✓ ¼ cup water
- ✓ 4 oz watercress

Directions:
- ❖ In a blender, add all ingredients and process until creamy and uniform.

Ingredients:
- ✓ 1 tsp low carb protein powder
- ✓ 1 tbsp chia seeds
- ✓ 1 tbsp unsweetened cocoa powder
- ✓ 4 fresh dates, pitted
- ❖ Chill and serve in glasses

Nutrition: Calories Calories 335; Fat: 31.7g Net Carbs: 12.7g, Protein: 7g

20) Special Bacon and Egg Quesadillas

Preparation Time: 30 minutes

Servings: 4

Ingredients:
- ✓ 8 low carb tortilla shells
- ✓ 6 eggs
- ✓ 1 cup water
- ✓ 3 tbsp butter

Directions:
- ❖ Bring the eggs to a boil in water over medium heat for 10 minutes. Transfer the eggs to an ice water bath, peel the shells, and chop them. Fry the bacon in a skillet over medium heat for 4 minutes until crispy. Remove and chop. Sauté the onion in the remaining grease 2 minutes; set aside.
- ❖ Melt 1 tbsp of butter in another skillet over medium heat. Lay one tortilla in a skillet and sprinkle with some Swiss cheese

Ingredients:
- ✓ 1 ½ cups grated cheddar cheese
- ✓ 1 ½ cups grated Swiss cheese
- ✓ 5 bacon slices
- ✓ 1 medium onion, thinly sliced
- ✓ 1 tbsp parsley, chopped
- ❖ Add some chopped eggs and bacon over the cheese, top with onion, and sprinkle with some cheddar cheese. Cover with another tortilla shell. Cook for 45 seconds
- ❖ Carefully flip the quesadilla, and cook the other side too for 45 seconds. Remove to a plate and repeat the cooking process using the remaining tortilla shells. Garnish with parsley and serve warm.

Nutrition: Calories Calories 449, Fat 48.7g, Net Carbs 6.8g, Protein 29.1g

21) Delicious Almond Waffles with Cinnamon Cream

Preparation Time: 25 minutes

Servings: 6

Ingredients:

- ✓ Cinnamon cream
- ✓ 8 oz cream cheese, softened
- ✓ 1 tsp cinnamon powder
- ✓ 3 tbsp swerve brown sugar
- ✓ 2 tbsp cinnamon

Directions:

- ❖ Combine cream cheese, cinnamon, and swerve with a mixer until smooth. Cover and chill until ready to use.
- ❖ To make the waffles, whisk the butter, milk, and eggs in a medium bowl. Add the stevia and baking powder and mix. Stir in the almond flour and combine until no lumps exist

Ingredients:

- ✓ Waffles
- ✓ 5 tbsp butter, melted
- ✓ 1 ½ cups unsweetened almond milk
- ✓ 7 large eggs
- ✓ ¼ tsp liquid stevia
- ✓ ½ tsp baking powder
- ✓ 1 ½ cups almond flour
- ❖ Let the batter sit for 5 minutes to thicken. Spritz a waffle iron with a cooking spray.
- ❖ Ladle a ¼ cup of the batter into the waffle iron and cook according to the manufacturer's instructions until golden, about 10 minutes in total. Repeat with the remaining batter. Slice the waffles into quarters. Apply the cinnamon spread in between each of two waffles and snap. Serve.

Nutrition: Calories Calories 307, Fat 24g, Net Carbs 8g, Protein 12g

22) Special Cajun Shrimp and Sausage Skillets

Preparation Time: 20 minutes

Servings: 2-4

Ingredients:

- ✓ 2 tablespoons avocado oil or ghee
- ✓ 12 oz andouille sausage, sliced
- ✓ 1 tbsp finely minced garlic
- ✓ 1 small red bell pepper, sliced
- ✓ 1 small green bell pepper, sliced
- ✓ salt and pepper to taste

Directions:

- ❖ Heat a large skillet over medium-high heat.
- ❖ Once the skillet is hot, add in the avocado oil or ghee.
- ❖ Add the minced garlic and cook for minute until fragrant.
- ❖ Add the sliced andouille sausage and cook for three to four minutes to brown on both sides.
- ❖ When the sausage has browned, add the sliced bell peppers and onions to the skillet.

Ingredients:

- ✓ 1 small orange bell pepper, sliced
- ✓ 1/2 yellow onion, sliced
- ✓ 1/4 cup sliced green onion
- ✓ 1 pound shrimp, peeled and deveined
- ✓ 1/2 tablespoon cajun seasoning (plus more to taste)
- ✓ juice of one lemon
- ❖ Season with salt, pepper, and the cajun seasoning. Cook the veggies for three to four minutes.
- ❖ Next, add the shrimp to the skillet and toss to combine.
- ❖ Cook for two to three minutes until the shrimp is translucent and cooked through.
- ❖ Remove the skillet from the heat and add the lemon juice, sliced green onion, and more seasoning to taste.
- ❖ Serve immediately.

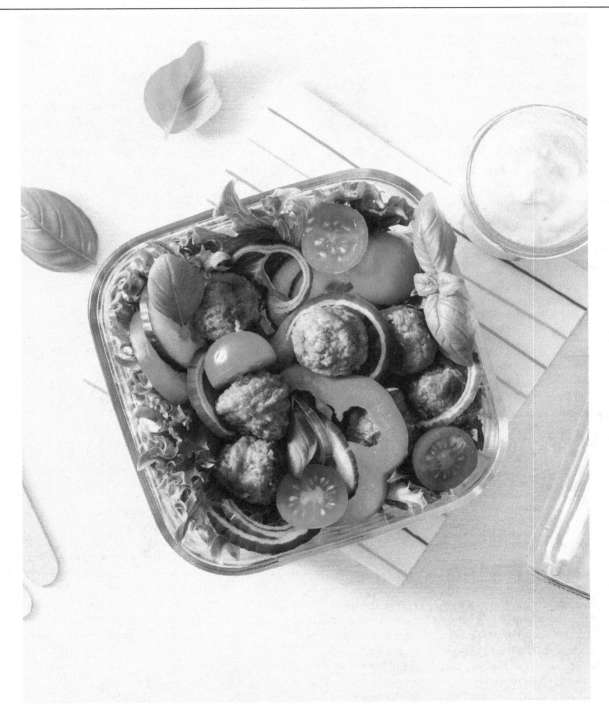

23) Special and Sweet Chili Grilled Chicken

Preparation Time: 30 minutes

Servings: 6

Ingredients:

- ✓ 2 lb chicken breasts
- ✓ 4 cloves garlic, minced
- ✓ 2 tbsp fresh oregano, chopped
- ✓ ½ cup lemon juice

Ingredients:

- ✓ 2/3 cup olive oil
- ✓ 1 tbsp erythritol
- ✓ Salt and black pepper to taste
- ✓ 3 small chilies, minced

Directions:

- ❖ Preheat grill to high heat. In a bowl, mix the garlic, oregano, lemon juice, olive oil, chilies, and erythritol. Cover the chicken with plastic wraps and use the rolling pin to pound to ½-inch thickness.

- ❖ Remove the wrap and brush the spice mixture on the chicken on all sides. Place on the grill and cook for 15 minutes, flip, and continue cooking for 10 more minutes. Remove to a plate and serve with salad.

Nutrition: Calories 265, Fat 9g, Net Carbs 3g, Protein 26g

24) Easy Chicken and Squash Traybake

Preparation Time: 50 minutes

Servings: 4

Ingredients:

- ✓ 1 ½ lb chicken thighs
- ✓ 1 lb butternut squash, cubed
- ✓ ½ cup black olives, pitted

Ingredients:

- ✓ ¼ cup olive oil
- ✓ 5 garlic cloves, sliced
- ✓ ¼ tbsp dried oregano

Directions:

- ❖ Preheat oven to 400°F. Place the chicken in a greased baking dish with the skin down. Place the garlic, olives, and butternut squash around the chicken.

- ❖ Drizzle with olive oil. Sprinkle with black pepper, salt, and oregano. Bake in the oven for 45 minutes until golden brown. Serve warm.

Nutrition: Calories: 411, Fat: 15g, Net Carbs: 5.5g, Protein: 31g

25) Bell Pepper and Beef Sausage Omelette

Preparation Time: approx. 60 minutes

Servings: 4

Ingredients:

- ✓ 12 whole eggs
- ✓ 1 cup sour cream
- ✓ 1 tbsp butter

Ingredients:

- ✓ 2 red bell peppers, chopped
- ✓ 12 oz ground beef sausage
- ✓ ¼ cup shredded cheddar

Directions:

- ❖ Preheat the oven to 350 F. Crack the eggs into a blender; add the sour cream, salt, and pepper. Process over low speed to mix the ingredients; set aside. Melt butter in a large skillet over medium heat. Add bell peppers and sauté until soft, 6 minutes; set aside. Add the beef sausage and cook until brown, continuously stirring and breaking the lumps into small bits, 10 minutes.

- ❖ Flatten the beef on the bottom of skillet, scatter bell peppers on top, pour the egg mixture all over, and scatter the top with cheddar cheese. Put the skillet in the oven and bake for 30 minutes or until the eggs set and the cheddar cheese melts. Remove, slice the frittata, and serve warm with a salad.

Nutrition: Calories 617; Net Carbs 5g; Fat 50g; Protein 33g

26) Italian Chili Zucchini Beef Lasagna

Preparation Time: approx. 55 minutes

Servings: 4

Ingredients:

- ✓ ½ cup Pecorino Romano cheese
- ✓ 4 yellow zucchini, sliced
- ✓ Salt and black pepper to taste
- ✓ 1 tbsp lard
- ✓ ½ lb ground beef
- ✓ 1 tsp garlic powder
- ✓ 1 tsp onion powder
- ✓ 2 tbsp coconut flour

Ingredients:

- ✓ 1 ½ cups grated mozzarella
- ✓ 2 cups crumbled goat cheese
- ✓ 1 large egg
- ✓ 2 cups marinara sauce
- ✓ 1 tbsp Italian herb seasoning
- ✓ ¼ tsp red chili flakes
- ✓ ¼ cup fresh basil leaves

Directions:

- ❖ Preheat oven to 375 F. Melt the lard in a skillet and cook beef for 10 minutes; set aside. In a bowl, combine garlic powder, onion powder, coconut flour, salt, pepper, mozzarella cheese, half of Pecorino cheese, goat cheese, and egg. Mix Italian herb seasoning and chili flakes with marinara sauce. Make a single layer of the zucchini in a greased baking dish, spread ¼ of the egg mixture on top, and ¼ of the marinara sauce.

- ❖ Repeat the process and top with the remaining Pecorino cheese. Bake in the oven for 20 minutes. Garnish with basil, slice, and serve.

Nutrition: Calories 608; Net Carbs 5.5g; Fat 37g; Protein 52g

27) Easy Tarragon Beef Meatloaf

Preparation Time: approx. 70 minutes

Servings: 4

Ingredients:

- ✓ 2 lb ground beef
- ✓ 3 tbsp flaxseed meal
- ✓ 2 large eggs
- ✓ 2 tbsp olive oil
- ✓ 1 lemon, zested

Ingredients:

- ✓ ¼ cup chopped tarragon
- ✓ ¼ cup chopped oregano
- ✓ 4 garlic cloves, minced

Directions:

- ❖ Preheat the oven to 400 F. Grease a loaf pan with cooking spray. In a bowl, combine beef, salt, pepper, and flaxseed meal; set aside. In another bowl, whisk the eggs with olive oil, lemon zest, tarragon, oregano, and garlic. Pour the mixture onto the beef mix and evenly combine.

- ❖ Spoon the meat mixture into the pan and press to fit in. Bake in oven for 1 hour. Remove the pan, tilt to drain the meat's liquid, and let cool for 5 minutes. Slice, garnish with some lemon slices, and serve with curried cauli rice.

Nutrition: Calories 631; Net Carbs 2.8g; Fat 38g; Protein 64g

28) Italian Broccoli Beef Bake with Pancetta

Preparation Time: approx. 55 minutes

Servings: 4

Ingredients:
- ✓ 1 large broccoli head, cut into florets
- ✓ 6 slices pancetta, chopped
- ✓ 2 tbsp olive oil
- ✓ 1 lb ground beef
- ✓ 2 tbsp butter

Ingredients:
- ✓ 1 cup coconut cream
- ✓ 2 oz cream cheese, softened
- ✓ 1 ¼ cups grated cheddar
- ✓ ¼ cup chopped scallions

Directions:
- ❖ Preheat the oven to 300 F. Fill a pot with water and bring to a boil. Pour in broccoli and blanch for 2 minutes. Drain and set aside. Place pancetta in the pot and fry for 5 minutes. Remove to a plate. Heat oil in the pot and cook the beef until brown for 5-6 minutes. Add in coconut cream, cream cheese, two-thirds of cheddar cheese, salt, and pepper and stir for 7 minutes.

- ❖ Arrange the broccoli florets in a baking dish, pour the beef mixture over, and scatter the top with pancetta and scallions. Bake in the oven until the cheese is bubbly and golden, 20 minutes. Top with the remaining cheddar and bake for 10 more minutes. Serve.

Nutrition: Calories 854; Net Carbs 7.3g; Fat 69g; Protein 51g

29) Slow-Cooking BBQ Beef Sliders

Preparation Time: approx. 12 hours 25 minutes

Servings: 4

Ingredients:
- ✓ 4 zero carb hamburger buns, halved
- ✓ 3 lb chuck roast, boneless
- ✓ 1 tsp onion powder
- ✓ 2 tsp garlic powder
- ✓ 1 tbsp smoked paprika
- ✓ 2 tbsp tomato paste

Ingredients:
- ✓ ¼ cup white vinegar
- ✓ 2 tbsp tamari sauce
- ✓ ½ cup bone broth
- ✓ ¼ cup melted butter
- ✓ Salt and black pepper to taste
- ✓ ¼ cup baby spinach
- ✓ 4 slices cheddar cheese

Directions:
- ❖ Cut the beef into two pieces. In a small bowl, combine salt, pepper, onion and garlic powders, and paprika. Rub the mixture onto beef and place it in a slow cooker. In another bowl, mix tomato paste, vinegar, tamari sauce, broth, and melted butter.

- ❖ Pour over the beef and cook for 4 hours on High. When the beef cooks, shred it using two forks. Divide the spinach between buns, spoon the meat on top, and add a cheddar cheese slice. Serve immediately.

Nutrition: Calories 648; Net Carbs 16g; Fat 27g; Protein 72g

30) Special .Roasted Beef Stacks with Cabbage

Preparation Time: approx. 55 minutes

Servings: 4

Ingredients:

- ✓ 1 head canon cabbage, shredded
- ✓ 1 lb chuck steak, sliced thinly across the grain
- ✓ 3 tbsp coconut flour

Ingredients:

- ✓ ¼ cup olive oil
- ✓ 1 tsp Italian mixed herb blend
- ✓ ½ cup bone broth
- ❖ Sprinkle the Italian herb blend and drizzle again with the remaining olive oil. Roast for 30 minutes. Remove the pan and carefully pour in the broth. Return to the oven and roast further for 10 minutes, until beef cooks through.

Directions:

- ❖ Preheat the oven to 400 F. In a zipper bag, add coconut flour, salt, and pepper. Mix and add the beef slices. Seal the bag and shake to coat. Make little mounds of cabbage. in a greased baking dish. Sprinkle with salt and pepper, and drizzle with some olive oil. Remove the beef strips from the coconut flour mixture, shake off the excess flour, and place 2-3 beef strips on each cabbage mound.

Nutrition: Calories 222; Net Carbs 1.5g; Fat 14g; Protein 18g

31) Easy Savory Portobello Beef Burgers

Preparation Time: approx. 30 minutes

Servings: 4

Ingredients:

- ✓ 4 large Portobello caps, destemmed and rinsed
- ✓ 1 lb ground beef
- ✓ Salt and black pepper to taste
- ✓ 1 tbsp Worcestershire sauce

Ingredients:

- ✓ 1 tbsp coconut oil
- ✓ 4 slices Monterey Jack
- ✓ 4 lettuce leaves
- ✓ 4 large tomato slices
- ✓ ¼ cup mayonnaise
- ❖ Remove to serving plates. Cook the beef patties in the skillet until brown, 10 minutes in total. Place the cheese slices on the beef, allow melting for 1 minute and lift each beef patty onto each mushroom cap. Cover with the lettuce, tomato slices, and mayo and serve.

Directions:

- ❖ In a bowl, combine beef, salt, pepper, and Worcestershire sauce. Using your hands, mold the meat into 4 patties, and set aside. Heat the coconut oil in a skillet over medium heat. Place in the Portobello caps and cook until softened, 4 minutes.

Nutrition: Calories 332; Net Carbs 0.7g; Fat 22g; Protein 29g

32) Rich Spicy Enchilada Beef Stuffed Peppers

Preparation Time: approx. 70 minutes

Servings: 6

Ingredients:

- ✓ 6 bell peppers, deseeded
- ✓ 1 ½ tbsp olive oil
- ✓ 3 tbsp butter, softened
- ✓ ½ white onion, chopped
- ✓ 3 cloves garlic, minced

Ingredients:

- ✓ 2 ½ lb ground beef
- ✓ 3 tsp enchilada seasoning
- ✓ 1 cup cauliflower rice
- ✓ ¼ cup grated cheddar cheese
- ✓ Sour cream for serving
- ❖ Spoon the mixture into the peppers, top with the cheddar cheese, and put the stuffed peppers in a greased baking dish. Bake for 40 minutes. Drop generous dollops of sour cream on the peppers and serve.

Directions:

- ❖ Preheat oven to 400 F. Melt butter in a skillet over medium heat and sauté onion and garlic for 3 minutes. Stir in beef, enchilada seasoning, salt, and pepper. Cook for 10 minutes. Mix in the cauli rice until well incorporated.

Nutrition: Calories 409; Net Carbs 4g; Fat 21g; Protein 45g

33) Simple Spicy Beef Lettuce Wraps

Preparation Time: approx. 20 minutes

Servings: 4

Ingredients:

- ✓ 1 lb chuck steak, sliced thinly against the grain
- ✓ 3 tbsp ghee, divided
- ✓ 1 large white onion, chopped
- ✓ 2 garlic cloves, minced
- ✓ 1 jalapeño pepper, chopped

Ingredients:

- ✓ 2 tsp red curry powder
- ✓ 1 cup cauliflower rice
- ✓ 8 small lettuce leaves
- ✓ ¼ cup sour cream for topping

- ❖ Lay out the lettuce leaves on a lean flat surface and spoon the beef mixture onto the middle part of them, 3 tbsp per leaf. Top with sour cream, wrap the leaves, and serve.

Directions:

- ❖ Melt 2 tbsp of ghee in a large deep skillet; season the beef and cook until brown and cooked within, 10 minutes; set aside. Sauté the onion for 3 minutes. Pour in garlic, salt, pepper, and jalapeño and cook for 1 minute.
- ❖ Add the remaining ghee, curry powder, and beef. Cook for 5 minutes and stir in the cauliflower rice. Sauté until adequately mixed and the cauliflower is slightly softened, 2 to 3 minutes. Adjust the taste with salt and black pepper.

Nutrition: Calories 298; Net Carbs 3.3g; Fat 18g; Protein 27g

34) Saturday Beef Sausage Pizza

Preparation Time: approx. 45 minutes

Servings: 4

Ingredients:

- ✓ 2 tbsp cream cheese, softened
- ✓ 6 oz shredded cheese
- ✓ ¾ cup almond flour
- ✓ 1 egg
- ✓ 1 tsp plain vinegar
- ✓ 2 tbsp butter

Ingredients:

- ✓ 8 oz ground beef sausage
- ✓ ¼ cup tomato sauce
- ✓ ½ tsp dried basil
- ✓ 4 ½ oz shredded mozzarella

Directions:

- ❖ Preheat oven to 400 F. Line a pizza pan with parchment paper. Melt cream and mozzarella cheeses in a skillet while stirring until evenly combined. Turn the heat off and mix in almond flour, egg, and vinegar. Let cool slightly.
- ❖ Flatten the mixture onto the pizza pan. Cover with another parchment paper and using a rolling pin, smoothen the dough into a circle. Take off the parchment paper on top, prick the dough all over with a fork and bake for 10 to 15 minutes until golden brown.

- ❖ While the crust bakes, melt butter in a skillet over and fry sausage until brown, 8 minutes. Turn the heat off. Spread the tomato sauce on the crust, top with basil, meat, and mozzarella cheese, and return to the oven. Bake for 12 minutes. Remove the pizza, slice, and serve warm.

Nutrition: Calories 361; Net Carbs 0.8g; Fat 21g; Protein 37g

35) Special Peanut Zucchini and Beef Pad Thai

Preparation Time: approx. 35 minutes

Servings: 4

Ingredients:

- ✓ 2 ½ lb chuck steak, sliced thinly against the grain
- ✓ 1 tsp crushed red pepper flakes
- ✓ 1 tsp freshly pureed garlic
- ✓ ¼ tsp freshly ground ginger
- ✓ Salt and black pepper to taste
- ✓ 2 tbsp peanut oil
- ✓ 3 large eggs, lightly beaten
- ✓ 1/3 cup beef broth

Ingredients:

- ✓ 3 ¼ tbsp peanut butter
- ✓ 2 tbsp tamari sauce
- ✓ 1 tbsp white vinegar
- ✓ ½ cup chopped green onions
- ✓ 2 garlic cloves, minced
- ✓ 4 zucchinis, spiralized
- ✓ ½ cup bean sprouts
- ✓ ½ cup crushed peanuts
- ❖ . Mix until adequately combined and simmer for 3 minutes. Stir in beef, zucchini, bean sprouts, and eggs. Cook for 1 minute. Garnish with peanuts.

Directions:

- ❖ In a bowl, combine garlic puree, ginger, salt, and pepper. Add in beef and toss to coat. Heat peanut oil in a deep skillet and cook the beef for 12 minutes; transfer to a plate. Pour the eggs to the skillet and scramble for 1 minute; set aside. Reduce the heat and combine broth, peanut butter, tamari sauce, vinegar, green onions, minced garlic, and red pepper flakes.

Nutrition: Calories 425; Net Carbs 3.3g; Fat 40g; Protein 70g

36) Hot Lemon and Spinach Cheeseburgers

Preparation Time: approx. 15 minutes

Servings: 4

Ingredients:

- ✓ 1 large tomato, sliced into 4 pieces and deseeded
- ✓ 1 lb ground beef
- ✓ ½ cup chopped cilantro
- ✓ 1 lemon, zested and juiced
- ✓ Salt and black pepper to taste
- ✓ 1 tsp garlic powder

Ingredients:

- ✓ 2 tbsp hot chili puree
- ✓ 16 large spinach leaves
- ✓ 4 tbsp mayonnaise
- ✓ 1 medium red onion, sliced
- ✓ ¼ cup grated Parmesan
- ✓ 1 avocado, halved, sliced
- ❖ Place a beef patty on each and spread 1 tbsp of mayo on top. Add a slice of tomato and onion, sprinkle with some Parmesan cheese, and place avocado on top. Cover with 2 pieces of spinach leaves each. Serve the burgers with cream cheese sauce.

Directions:

- ❖ Preheat the grill on high heat. In a bowl, add beef, cilantro, lemon zest, juice, salt, pepper, garlic powder, and chili puree. Mix the ingredients until evenly combined. Make 4 patties from the mixture. Grill for 3 minutes on each side. Transfer to a serving plate. Lay 2 spinach leaves side to side in 4 portions on a clean flat surface.

Nutrition: Calories 310; Net Carbs 6.5g; Fat 16g; Protein 29g

37) Easy Herby Beef Meatballs

Preparation Time: approx. 30 minutes

Servings: 4

Ingredients:

- ✓ 1 lb ground beef
- ✓ 1 red onion, finely chopped
- ✓ 2 red bell peppers, chopped
- ✓ 2 garlic cloves, minced
- ✓ 2 tbsp melted butter

Ingredients:

- ✓ 1 tsp dried basil
- ✓ 2 tbsp tamari sauce
- ✓ Salt and black pepper to taste
- ✓ 1 tbsp dried rosemary
- ✓ 1 tbsp olive oil

Directions:

- ❖ Preheat the oven to 400 F. In a bowl, mix beef, onion, bell peppers, garlic, butter, basil, tamari sauce, salt, pepper, and rosemary. Form 1-inch meatballs from the mixture and place on a greased baking sheet.
- ❖ Drizzle olive oil over the beef and bake in the oven for 20 minutes or until the meatballs brown on the outside. Serve garnished with scallions and topped with ranch dressing.

Nutrition: Calories 618; Net Carbs 2.5g; Fat 33g; Protein 74g

38) Paleo and .Keto Burgers

Preparation Time: approx. 15 minutes

Servings: 4

Ingredients:

- ✓ 1 pound ground beef
- ✓ ½ tsp onion powder
- ✓ ½ tsp garlic powder
- ✓ 2 tbsp ghee
- ✓ 1 tsp Dijon mustard

Directions:

- ❖ Mix together beef, onion powder, garlic powder, and mustard in a bowl. Create 4 burgers.

Ingredients:

- ✓ 4 zero carb burger buns
- ✓ ¼ cup mayonnaise
- ✓ 1 tsp Sriracha sauce
- ✓ 4 tbsp coleslaw
- ✓ Salt and black pepper to taste
- ❖ Melt ghee in a skillet and cook the burgers for 3 minutes per side. Serve on buns topped with mayonnaise, sriracha sauce, and coleslaw.

Nutrition: Calories 664; Net Carbs 7.9g; Fat 55g; Protein 39g

39) Special Beef Taco pizza

Preparation Time: approx. 45 minutes

Servings: 4

Ingredients:

- ✓ 2 cups shredded mozzarella
- ✓ 2 tbsp cream cheese, softened
- ✓ 1 egg
- ✓ ¾ cup almond flour
- ✓ 1 lb ground beef
- ✓ 2 tsp taco seasoning
- ✓ ½ cup cheese sauce

Directions:

- ❖ Preheat oven to 390 F. Line a pizza pan with parchment paper. Microwave the mozzarella and cream cheeses for 1 minute. Remove and mix in egg and almond flour. Spread the mixture on the pan and bake for 15 minutes. Put the beef in a pot and cook for 5 minutes. Stir in taco seasoning.

Ingredients:

- ✓ 1 cup grated cheddar cheese
- ✓ 1 cup chopped lettuce
- ✓ 1 tomato, diced
- ✓ ¼ cup sliced black olives
- ✓ 1 cup sour cream for topping

- ❖ Spread the cheese sauce on the crust and top with the meat. Add cheddar cheese, lettuce, tomato, and black olives. Bake until the cheese melts, 5 minutes. Remove the pizza, drizzle sour cream on top, and serve.

Nutrition: Calories 590; Net Carbs 7.9g; Fat 29g; Protein 64g

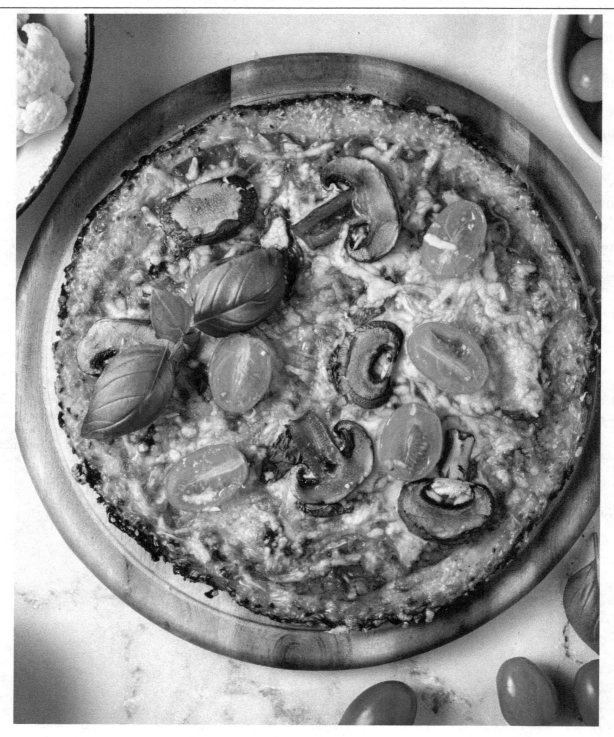

40) Tofu Nuggets with cilantro sauce

Preparation Time: 25 minutes

Servings: 4

Ingredients:
- ✓ 1 lime, ½ squeezed and ½ cut into wedges
- ✓ 1 ½ cups olive oil
- ✓ 28 ounces tofu, pressed and diced
- ✓ 1 egg, lightly beaten
- ✓ 1 cup golden flax seed meal

Directions:
- ❖ Heat the olive oil in a deep skillet. Coat the tofu cubes in the egg and then in the flaxseed meal. Fry until golden brown.

Ingredients:
- ✓ 1 ripe avocado, chopped
- ✓ ½ tbsp chopped cilantro
- ✓ Salt and black pepper to taste
- ✓ ½ tbsp olive oil

- ❖ Transfer to a plate. Place the avocado, cilantro, salt, pepper and lime juice in a blender; blend until smooth. Pour into a bowl, add the tofu nuggets and lime wedges to serve.

Nutrition: Calories 665; Net carbs 6.2g, fat 54g, protein 32g

41) Spicy Brussels sprouts with carrots

Preparation Time: 15 minutes

Servings: 4

Ingredients:
- ✓ 1 pound Brussels sprouts
- ✓ ¼ cup olive oil
- ✓ 4 green onions, chopped

Directions:
- ❖ Sauté green onions in hot olive oil for 2 minutes. Sprinkle with salt and pepper and transfer to a plate. Cut the Brussels sprouts and split them in half.

Ingredients:
- ✓ 2 carrots, grated
- ✓ Salt and black pepper to taste
- ✓ Hot chili sauce
- ❖ Leave the small ones as whole. Pour the Brussels sprouts and carrots into the same saucepan and sauté until softened but al dente. Season to taste and toss with the onions. Cook for 3 minutes. Add chili sauce and serve.

Nutrition: Calories 198; Net carbohydrates 6.5g; Fat 14g; Protein 4.9g

42) Zucchini-Cranberry Cake Squares

Preparation Time: 45 minutes

Servings: 6

Ingredients:
- ✓ 1 ¼ cups chopped zucchini
- ✓ 2 tbsp olive oil
- ✓ ½ cup dried cranberries
- ✓ 1 lemon, peeled
- ✓ 3 eggs

Directions:
- ❖ Preheat oven to 350 F. Line a square cake pan with baking paper. Combine the zucchini, olive oil, cranberries, lemon zest and eggs in a bowl until evenly combined.

Ingredients:
- ✓ 1 ½ cups almond flour
- ✓ ½ tsp baking powder
- ✓ 1 tsp cinnamon powder
- ✓ A pinch of salt

- ❖ Add the almond flour, baking powder, cinnamon powder and salt into the mixture. Pour the mixture into the cake pan and bake for 30 minutes. Remove from the oven, let cool in the cake pan for 10 minutes and transfer the cake to a wire rack to cool completely. Cut into squares and serve.

Nutrition: Calories 121; Net Carbs 2.5g, Fat 10g, Protein 4g

43) Fried rice egg with grilled cheese

Preparation Time: 10 minutes

Servings: 4

Ingredients:

- ✓ 2 cups cauliflower rice, steamed
- ✓ ½ pound halloumi, cut into ¼- to ½-inch slabs
- ✓ 1 tbsp ghee
- ✓ 4 eggs, beaten

Directions:

- ❖ Melt the ghee in a skillet and pour in the eggs. Rotate the pan to scatter the eggs and cook for 1 minute. Move the scrambled eggs to the side of the skillet, add the bell bell pepper and green beans and saute for 3 minutes. Pour in the cauli rice and cook for 2 minutes.

Ingredients:

- ✓ 1 green bell pepper, chopped
- ✓ ¼ cup green beans, chopped
- ✓ 1 tsp soy sauce
- ✓ 2 tbsp chopped parsley
- ❖ Add the soy sauce; combine evenly and cook for 2 minutes. Distribute to plates, garnish with parsley and set aside. Preheat a grill pan and grill halloumi cheese on both sides until cheese turns slightly brown. Place on the side of the rice and serve hot.

Nutrition: Calories 275; Net carbs 4.5g, fat 19g, protein 15g

44) Fake Mushroom Risotto

Preparation Time: 15 minutes

Servings: 4

Ingredients:

- ✓ 2 shallots, diced
- ✓ 3 tbsp olive oil
- ✓ ¼ cup vegetable stock
- ✓ ⅓ cup Parmesan cheese

Directions:

- ❖ Heat 2 tbsp oil in a saucepan, add mushrooms and cook over medium heat for 3 minutes.

Ingredients:

- ✓ 4 tbsp butter
- ✓ 3 tbsp chopped chives
- ✓ 2 pounds mushrooms, sliced
- ✓ 4 1/2 cups rinsed cauliflower
- ❖ Remove and set aside. Heat the remaining oil and cook the shallots for 2 minutes. Add the cauliflower and broth and cook until the liquid is absorbed. Stir in the rest of the ingredients.

Nutrition: Calories 264; Net carbs 8.4g; Fat 18g; Protein 11g

45) Eggplant pizza with cheese

Preparation Time: 40 minutes

Servings: 2

Ingredients:

- ✓ 6 ounces grated mozzarella cheese
- ✓ 2 tbsp cream cheese
- ✓ 2 tbsp Parmesan cheese
- ✓ 1 tsp oregano
- ✓ ½ cup almond flour
- ✓ 2 tbsp psyllium husk

Directions:

- ❖ Preheat oven to 400 F. Melt the mozzarella cheese in the microwave. Combine cream cheese, Parmesan cheese, oregano, almond flour and psyllium husk in a bowl. Add the melted mozzarella cheese and stir to combine.

Ingredients:

- ✓ 4 ounces grated cheddar cheese
- ✓ ¼ cup marinara sauce
- ✓ Eggplant, sliced
- ✓ 1 tomato, sliced
- ✓ 2 tbsp chopped basil
- ✓ 6 black olives
- ❖ Divide the dough into 2. Roll out the crusts into circles and place on a lined baking sheet. Bake for 10 minutes. Add the cheddar cheese, marinara, eggplant, tomato and basil. Return to oven and bake for 10 minutes. Serve with olives.

Nutrition: Calories 510; Net Carbs 3.7g; Fat 39g; Protein 31g

46) Eggplant and Goat Cheese Pizza

Preparation Time: 45 minutes

Servings: 4

Ingredients:
- ✓ 4 tbsp olive oil
- ✓ 2 eggplants, sliced lengthwise
- ✓ 1 cup tomato sauce
- ✓ 2 garlic cloves, minced
- ✓ 1 red onion, sliced
- ✓ 12 ounces goat cheese, crumbled

Ingredients:
- ✓ Salt and black pepper to taste
- ✓ ½ tsp cinnamon powder
- ✓ 1 cup mozzarella cheese, shredded
- ✓ 2 tbsp oregano, chopped

Directions:
- ❖ Line a baking sheet with baking paper. Arrange eggplant slices on baking sheet and drizzle with a little olive oil. Bake for 20 minutes at 390 F. Heat the remaining olive oil in a skillet and sauté the garlic and onion for 3 minutes.

- ❖ Add goat cheese and tomato sauce and season with salt and pepper. Simmer for 10 minutes. Remove eggplant from oven and spread cheese sauce on top. Sprinkle with mozzarella cheese and oregano. Bake for 10 minutes more until cheese melts. Cut into slices and serve.

Nutrition: Calories 557; Net Carbs 8.3g; Fat 44g; Protein 33g

47) Mushroom and broccoli pizza

Preparation Time: 25 minutes

Servings: 4

Ingredients:
- ✓ ½ cup almond flour
- ✓ ¼ tsp salt
- ✓ 2 tbsp ground psyllium husk
- ✓ 2 tbsp olive oil
- ✓ 1 cup fresh sliced mushrooms
- ✓ 1 white onion, thinly sliced

Ingredients:
- ✓ 3 cups broccoli florets
- ✓ 2 cloves garlic, minced
- ✓ ½ cup unsweetened pizza sauce
- ✓ 4 tomatoes, sliced
- ✓ 1 ½ cups mozzarella cheese, grated
- ✓ ⅓ cup grated Parmesan cheese

Directions:
- ❖ Preheat oven to 390 F. Line a baking sheet with parchment paper. In a bowl, mix almond flour, salt, psyllium powder, 1 tbsp olive oil and 1 cup warm water until a dough forms. Spread the dough onto the pizza pan and bake for 10 minutes.

- ❖ Heat the remaining olive oil in a skillet and sauté mushrooms, onion, garlic and broccoli for 5 minutes. Spread the pizza sauce over the crust and top with the broccoli mixture, tomato, mozzarella and Parmesan. Bake for 5 minutes. Serve in slices.

Nutrition: Calories 180; Net carbs 3.6g; Fat 9g; Protein 17g

48) Tofu radish bowls

Preparation Time: 35 minutes

Ingredients:
- ¼ cup baby mushrooms, chopped
- 2 yellow peppers, chopped
- 1 block of tofu (14 oz), cubed
- 1 tbsp + 1 tbsp olive oil
- 1 ½ cups shredded radishes

Directions:
- Heat 1 tbsp olive oil in a skillet and add tofu, radishes, onions, mushrooms and peppers; cook for 10 minutes. Divide among 4 bowls. Heat the remaining oil in the skillet, crack an egg into the pan and cook until the white sets but the yolk is quite runny.

Ingredients:
- ½ cup chopped white onions
- 4 eggs
- 1/3 cup tomato sauce
- A handful of chopped parsley
- 1 avocado, and chopped
- Transfer to the top of a bowl of tofu hash and make the remaining eggs. Top the bowls with the tomato sauce, parsley and avocado. Serve.

Nutrition: Calories 353; Net Carbs 5.9g, Fat 25g, Protein 19g

49) Tomato & Mozzarella Caprese Bake

Preparation Time: 25 minutes

Servings: 4

Ingredients:
- 4 tbsp olive oil
- 4 tomatoes, sliced
- 1 cup fresh mozzarella, sliced

Directions:
- In a baking dish, arrange the tomatoes and mozzarella slices. In a bowl, mix the pesto, mayonnaise and half of the Parmesan cheese; stir to combine.

Ingredients:
- 2 tbsp basil pesto
- 1 cup mayonnaise
- 2 ounces Parmesan cheese, grated
- Spread this mixture over the tomatoes and mozzarella and top with the remaining Parmesan cheese. Bake for 20 minutes at 360 F. Remove, let cool slightly and slice to serve.

Nutrition: Calories 420; Net Carbs 4.9g; Fat 36g; Protein 17g

50) Cookies with heart of pistachio

Preparation Time: 30 min + cooling time

Servings: 4

Ingredients:
- 1 cup butter, softened
- 2/3 cup sugar swerve
- 1 large egg, beaten
- 2 tsp pistachio extract

Directions:
- Add the butter and swerve sugar to a bowl and beat until smooth and creamy. Beat in the egg until combined. Stir in the pistachio extract and almond flour until a smooth dough forms. Wrap the dough in plastic wrap and chill for 10 minutes. Preheat oven to 350 F. Lightly dust a cutting board with almond flour. Unroll the dough and roll it out to a thickness of 2 inches.

Ingredients:
- 2 cups almond flour
- ½ cup dark chocolate
- 2 tbsp chopped pistachios

- Cut out as many cookies as you can get, while rolling back the scraps to make more cookies. Place the cookies on the baking sheet lined with parchment paper and bake for 15 minutes. Transfer to a wire rack to cool completely. Melt the dark chocolate in the microwave. Dip one side of each cookie into the melted chocolate. Garnish chocolate side with pistachios and let cool on a wire rack. Serve.

Nutrition: Calories 470; Net carbs 3.4g, fat 45g, protein 6.2g

51) Avocado and tomato burritos

Preparation Time: 10 minutes

Ingredients:
- ✓ 2 cups cauli rice
- ✓ 6 low carb tortillas
- ✓ 2 cups sour cream sauce

Directions:
- ❖ Pour cauli rice into a bowl, sprinkle with a little water, and microwave for 2 minutes to soften. On the tortillas, spread the sour cream and spread the salsa on top.

Nutrition: Calories 303, Fat 25g, Net Carbs 6g, Protein 8g

Servings: 4

Ingredients:
- ✓ 1 ½ cups herbed tomato sauce
- ✓ 2 avocados, peeled, pitted and sliced

- ❖ Top with the cauli rice and spread the avocado evenly on top. Fold and tuck the burritos and cut in half. Serve.

52) Creamy cucumber and avocado soup

Preparation Time: 15 minutes

Ingredients:
- ✓ 4 large cucumbers, seeded and cut into pieces
- ✓ 1 large avocado, peeled and cut in half
- ✓ Salt and black pepper to taste
- ✓ 1 tbsp fresh cilantro, chopped
- ✓ 3 tbsp olive oil

Directions:
- ❖ Pour cucumbers, avocado halves, salt, black pepper, olive oil, lime juice, cilantro, 2 cups water and garlic into food processor. Puree the ingredients for 2 minutes or until smooth.

Nutrition: Calories 170, Fat 7.4g, Net Carbs 4.1g, Protein 3.7g

Servings: 4

Ingredients:
- ✓ 2 limes, squeezed
- ✓ 2 tbsp minced garlic
- ✓ 2 tomatoes, chopped
- ✓ 1 avocado, chopped for garnish

- ❖ Pour mixture into a bowl and top with avocado and chopped tomatoes. Serve cold with zero carb bread.

53) Cauliflower "couscous" with lemon and Halloumi

Preparation Time: 5 minutes

Ingredients:
- ✓ 4 ounces of halloumi, sliced
- ✓ 2 tbsp olive oil
- ✓ 1 head of cauliflower, cut into florets
- ✓ ¼ cup chopped cilantro

Directions:
- ❖ Heat the olive oil in a skillet over medium heat. Add halloumi and fry for 2 minutes on each side until golden brown; set aside. Pour the cauli florets into a food processor and pulse until it crumbles and resembles couscous. Transfer to a bowl and steam in the microwave for 2 minutes.

Nutrition: Calories 185, Fat 15.6g, Net Carbs 2.1g, Protein 12g

Servings: 4

Ingredients:
- ✓ ¼ cup chopped parsley
- ✓ ¼ cup chopped mint
- ✓ ½ lemon, squeezed
- ✓ Salt and black pepper to taste
- ✓ 1 avocado, sliced for garnish

- ❖ Remove the bowl from the microwave and allow the cauli to cool. Add the cilantro, parsley, mint, lemon juice, salt and pepper. Top the couscous with avocado slices and serve with grilled halloumi and vegetable sauce.

54) Zucchini lasagna with ricotta cheese and spinach

Preparation Time: 50 minutes

Servings: 4

Ingredients:

- ✓ 2 zucchini, sliced
- ✓ Salt and black pepper to taste
- ✓ 2 cups ricotta cheese

Directions:

- ❖ Preheat oven to 370°F. Place zucchini slices in a colander and sprinkle with salt. Let stand and drain liquid for 5 minutes and pat dry with paper towels. Mix the ricotta, mozzarella, salt and black pepper to combine evenly and spread ¼ cup of the mixture over the bottom of the baking dish.
- ❖ Arrange ⅓ of the zucchini slices on top, spread 1 cup of the tomato sauce, and scatter ⅓ cup of the spinach on top.

Ingredients:

- ✓ 2 cups shredded mozzarella cheese
- ✓ 3 cups tomato sauce
- ✓ 1 cup spinach
- ❖ Repeat the layering process two more times to run out of ingredients, finally making sure to layer with the last ¼ cup of cheese mixture.
- ❖ Grease one end of the aluminum foil with cooking spray and cover the baking sheet with the foil. Bake for 35 minutes, remove the foil and bake further for 5-10 minutes or until the cheese has a nice golden brown color. Remove dish, let rest for 5 minutes, make lasagna slices and serve warm.

55) Briam with tomato sauce

Preparation Time: 40 minutes

Servings: 4

Ingredients:

- ✓ 3 tbsp olive oil
- ✓ 1 large eggplant, halved and sliced
- ✓ 1 large onion, thinly sliced
- ✓ 3 garlic cloves, sliced
- ✓ 2 tomatoes, diced
- ✓ 1 rutabaga, diced

Directions:

- ❖ Preheat oven to 400°F. Heat the olive oil in a skillet over medium heat and fry the eggplant and zucchini slices for 6 minutes until golden brown. Remove them to a casserole dish and arrange them in a single layer.

Ingredients:

- ✓ 1 cup unsweetened tomato sauce
- ✓ 4 zucchini, sliced
- ✓ ¼ cup water
- ✓ Salt and black pepper to taste
- ✓ ¼ tsp dried oregano
- ✓ 2 tbsp fresh parsley, chopped
- ❖ Sauté the onion and garlic in the oil for 3 minutes. Remove to a bowl. Add the tomatoes, rutabaga, tomato sauce and water and mix well. Stir in salt, pepper, oregano and parsley. Pour the mixture over the eggplant and zucchini. Place the dish in the oven and bake for 25-30 minutes. Serve the briam hot.

Nutrition: Calories Calories 365, Fat 12g, Net Carbohydrates 12.5g, Protein 11.3g

56) Creamy vegetable stew

Preparation Time: 25 minutes

Servings: 4

Ingredients:
- ✓ 2 tbsp ghee
- ✓ 1 tbsp onion and garlic puree
- ✓ 2 medium carrots, shredded
- ✓ 1 head of cauliflower, cut into florets

Ingredients:
- ✓ 2 cups green beans, cut in half
- ✓ Salt and black pepper to taste
- ✓ 1 cup water
- ✓ 1 ½ cups heavy cream
- ❖ Pour in water, stir again and cook over low heat for 15 minutes. Stir in the heavy cream to incorporate and turn off the heat. Serve the stew with almond flour bread.

Directions:
- ❖ Melt ghee in a saucepan over medium heat and sauté onion and garlic puree to be fragrant, 2 minutes. Stir in carrots, cauliflower and green beans for 5 minutes. Season with salt and black pepper.

Nutrition: Calories 310, fat 26.4g, net carbs 6g, protein 8g

57) Tempeh kabobs with vegetables

Preparation Time: 30 minutes + cooling time

Servings: 4

Ingredients:
- ✓ 2 tbsp ghee
- ✓ 1 tbsp onion and garlic puree
- ✓ 2 medium carrots, shredded
- ✓ 1 head of cauliflower, cut into florets

Ingredients:
- ✓ 2 cups green beans, cut in half
- ✓ Salt and black pepper to taste
- ✓ 1 cup water
- ✓ 1 ½ cups heavy cream
- ❖ Pour in water, stir again and cook over low heat for 15 minutes. Stir in the heavy cream to incorporate and turn off the heat. Serve the stew with almond flour bread.

Directions:
- ❖ Melt ghee in a saucepan over medium heat and sauté onion and garlic puree to be fragrant, 2 minutes. Stir in carrots, cauliflower and green beans for 5 minutes. Season with salt and black pepper.

Nutrition: Calories Calories 228, Fat 15g, Net Carbohydrates 3.6g, Protein 13.2g

58) Tempeh kabobs with vegetables

Preparation Time: 30 minutes + cooling time

Servings: 4

Ingredients:
- ✓ 1 yellow bell pepper, cut into pieces
- ✓ 10 ounces tempeh, cut into pieces
- ✓ 1 red onion, cut into pieces

Ingredients:
- ✓ 1 red bell bell pepper, cut into pieces
- ✓ 2 tbsp olive oil
- ✓ 1 cup unsweetened barbecue sauce
- ❖ Preheat grill to 350°F. Thread the tempeh, yellow bell pepper, red bell pepper and onion onto skewers. Brush the grill grate with olive oil, place the skewers on and brush with the barbecue sauce. Cook skewers for 3 minutes on each side, rotating and brushing with more barbecue sauce. Serve.

Directions:
- ❖ Bring the 1 ½ cups of water to a boil in a pot over medium heat, and once it's cooked, turn off the heat and add the tempeh. Cover the pot and allow the tempeh to steam for 5 minutes to remove the bitterness. Drain. Pour barbecue sauce into a bowl, add tempeh and coat with sauce. Refrigerate for 2 hours.

Nutrition: Calories Calories 228, Fat 15g, Net Carbohydrates 3.6g, Protein 13.2g

59) Cauliflower and Gouda Cheese Casserole

Preparation Time: 25 minutes

Servings: 4

Ingredients:

- ✓ 2 heads of cauliflower, cut into florets
- ✓ 2 tbsp olive oil
- ✓ 2 tbsp melted butter
- ✓ 1 white onion, chopped

Directions:

- ❖ Preheat oven to 350°F. Place cauli florets in a large microwave-safe bowl. Sprinkle with a little water and steam in the microwave for 4 to 5 minutes. Heat the olive oil in a saucepan over medium heat and sauté the onion for 3 minutes. Add the cauliflower, season with salt and pepper and stir in the almond milk.

Ingredients:

- ✓ Salt and black pepper to taste
- ✓ ¼ cup almond milk
- ✓ ½ cup almond flour
- ✓ 1 ½ cups gouda cheese, grated
- ❖ Cook over low heat for 3 minutes. Mix the melted butter with the almond flour. Stir in the cauliflower and half of the cheese. Sprinkle the top with the remaining cheese and bake for 10 minutes until the cheese is melted and golden brown on top. Plate the oven and serve with the salad.

Nutrition: Calories 215, Fat 15g, Net Carbs 4g, Protein 12g

60) Roasted Asparagus with Spicy Eggplant Sauce

Preparation Time: 35 minutes

Servings: 6

Ingredients:

- ✓ 1 ½ pounds asparagus, chopped
- ✓ ¼ cup + 2 tbsp olive oil
- ✓ ½ tsp paprika
- ✓ Eggplant Sauce
- ✓ 1 pound of eggplant
- ✓ ½ cup shallots, chopped

Directions:

- ❖ Preheat oven to 390°F. Line a parchment paper on a baking sheet. Add the asparagus. Season with 2 tbsp olive oil, paprika, black pepper and salt. Roast until cooked through, 9 minutes. Remove.
- ❖ Place the eggplant on a cookie sheet lined baking sheet. Bake in the oven for about 20 minutes.

Ingredients:

- ✓ 2 cloves garlic, minced
- ✓ 1 tbsp fresh lemon juice
- ✓ ½ tsp chili pepper
- ✓ Salt and black pepper to taste
- ✓ ¼ cup fresh cilantro, chopped

- ❖ Allow eggplant to cool. Peel them and discard the stems. Heat the remaining olive oil in a skillet over medium heat and add the garlic and shallots. Sauté for 3 minutes until tender.
- ❖ In a food processor, put together the black pepper, roasted eggplant, salt, lemon juice, shallot mixture, and red pepper. Add the cilantro and serve alongside the roasted asparagus spears.

Nutrition: Calories 149; Fat: 12.1g, Net Carbohydrates: 9g, Protein: 3.6g

61) Cook the squash

Preparation Time: 45 minutes

Servings: 6

Ingredients:

- ✓ 3 large pumpkins, peeled and sliced
- ✓ 1 cup almond flour
- ✓ 1 cup grated mozzarella cheese

Directions:

- ❖ Preheat oven to 350°F. Arrange the squash slices in a baking dish and drizzle with olive oil.

Ingredients:

- ✓ 3 tbsp olive oil
- ✓ ½ cup fresh parsley, chopped

- ❖ Bake for 35 minutes. Mix almond flour, mozzarella cheese and parsley and pour over squash. Return to oven and bake for another 5 minutes until top is golden brown. Serve warm.

Nutrition: Calories 125, Fat 4.8g, Net Carbs 5.7g, Protein 2.7g

62) Cremini Mushroom Stroganoff

Preparation Time: 25 minutes   **Servings: 4**

Ingredients:

- ✓ 3 tbsp butter
- ✓ 1 white onion, chopped
- ✓ 4 cups cremini mushrooms, diced

Directions:

- ❖ Melt the butter in a saucepan over medium heat and sauté the onion for 3 minutes until soft. Add the mushrooms and cook until tender, about 5 minutes. Add 2 cups of water and bring to a boil.

Ingredients:

- ✓ ½ cup heavy cream
- ✓ ½ cup Parmesan cheese, grated
- ✓ 1 ½ tbsp dried mixed herbs
- ❖ Cook for 10-15 minutes until the water reduces slightly. Pour in the heavy cream and Parmesan cheese. Stir to dissolve the cheese. Add the dried herbs and season. Simmer for 5 minutes. Serve hot.

Nutrition: Calories 284, Fat 28g, Net Carbs 1.5g, Protein 8g

63) Portobello Mushroom Burger

Preparation Time: 15 minutes   **Servings: 4**

Ingredients:

- ✓ 8 large portobello mushroom caps
- ✓ 1 minced garlic clove
- ✓ ½ cup of mayonnaise
- ✓ ½ tsp salt
- ✓ 4 tbsp olive oil
- ✓ ½ cup roasted red peppers, sliced

Directions:

- ❖ Preheat a grill over medium-high heat. In a bowl, crush the garlic with the salt using the back of a spoon. Stir in half the oil and brush the mushrooms and halloumi cheese with the mixture.
- ❖ Place the "sandwiches" on the skillet and grill them on both sides for 8 minutes until tender.

Ingredients:

- ✓ 2 medium tomatoes, chopped
- ✓ 4 halloumi slices, half-inch thick
- ✓ 1 tbsp red wine vinegar
- ✓ 2 tbsp Kalamata olives, chopped
- ✓ ½ tsp dried oregano
- ✓ 2 cups spinach
- ❖ Add the halloumi cheese slices to the grill. Cook for 2 minutes per side or until golden brown marks appear on the grill.
- ❖ In a bowl, mix red peppers, tomatoes, olives, vinegar, oregano, spinach and remaining olive oil; toss to coat. Spread mayonnaise on 4 mushroom "sandwiches", top with a slice of halloumi, a scoop of greens and top with remaining mushrooms. Serve and enjoy!

Nutrition: Calories 339, Fat 29.4g, Net Carbs 3.5g, Protein 10g

64) Sriracha tofu with yogurt sauce

Preparation Time: 40 minutes   **Servings: 4**

Ingredients:

- ✓ 12 ounces tofu, pressed and sliced
- ✓ 1 cup green onions, chopped
- ✓ 1 clove garlic, minced
- ✓ 2 tbsp vinegar
- ✓ 1 tbsp sriracha sauce
- ✓ 2 tbsp olive oil

Directions:

- ❖ Place the tofu slices, garlic, sriracha sauce, vinegar and green onions in a bowl. Let stand for 30 minutes. Place a nonstick skillet over medium heat and add oil to heat. Cook the tofu for 5 minutes until golden brown.

Ingredients:

- ✓ Yogurt Sauce
- ✓ 2 cloves garlic, crushed
- ✓ 2 tbsp fresh lemon juice
- ✓ Salt and black pepper to taste
- ✓ 1 tsp fresh dill
- ✓ 1 cup Greek yogurt
- ✓ 1 cucumber, shredded
- ❖ To make the sauce: In a bowl, mix garlic, salt, yogurt, black pepper, lemon juice and dill. Add shredded cucumber while stirring to combine. Serve tofu with a spoonful of yogurt sauce.

Nutrition: Calories 351; Fat: 25.9g, Net Carbohydrates: 8.1g, Protein: 17.5g

65) Jalapeño and Vegetable Stew

Preparation Time: 40 minutes   **Servings: 4**

Ingredients:

- ✓ 2 tbsp butter
- ✓ 1 cup leeks, chopped
- ✓ 1 clove garlic, minced
- ✓ ½ cup celery stalks, chopped
- ✓ ½ cup carrots, chopped
- ✓ 1 green bell bell pepper, chopped
- ✓ 1 jalapeño bell pepper, chopped
- ✓ 1 zucchini, chopped

Directions:

- ❖ Melt the butter in a saucepan over medium heat. Add the garlic and leeks and sauté for 3 minutes until soft and translucent. Add the celery, mushrooms, zucchini and carrots and sauté for another 5 minutes.

Ingredients:

- ✓ 1 cup mushrooms, sliced
- ✓ 1 ½ cups vegetable broth
- ✓ 2 tomatoes, chopped
- ✓ 2 tbsp fresh parsley, chopped
- ✓ 2 bay leaves
- ✓ Salt and black pepper to taste
- ✓ 1 tbsp vinegar
- ❖ Stir in the rest of the ingredients. Season with salt and pepper. Bring to a boil and simmer for 15-20 minutes or until cooked through. Divide among individual bowls and serve hot.

Nutrition: Calories 65; Fat: 2.7g, Net Carbohydrates: 9g, Protein: 2.7g

66) Raspberry and turmeric panna cotta

Preparation Time: 10 minutes + cooling time   **Servings: 6**

Ingredients:

- ✓ ½ tbsp unflavored vegetable gelatin powder
- ✓ 2 cups of coconut cream
- ✓ ¼ tsp vanilla extract
- ✓ 1 tsp turmeric

Directions:

- ❖ Mix the gelatin and ½ tbsp water and let it dissolve. Pour the coconut cream, vanilla extract, turmeric and erythritol into a saucepan and bring to a boil; simmer for 2 minutes. Turn off the heat. Stir in gelatin.

Ingredients:

- ✓ 1 tbsp erythritol
- ✓ 1 tbsp chopped toasted pecans
- ✓ 12 fresh raspberries
- ❖ Pour into 6 glasses, cover with plastic wrap and refrigerate for 2 hours. Top with pecans and raspberries and serve.

Nutrition: Calories 270; Net Carbs 3g; Fat 27g; Protein 4g

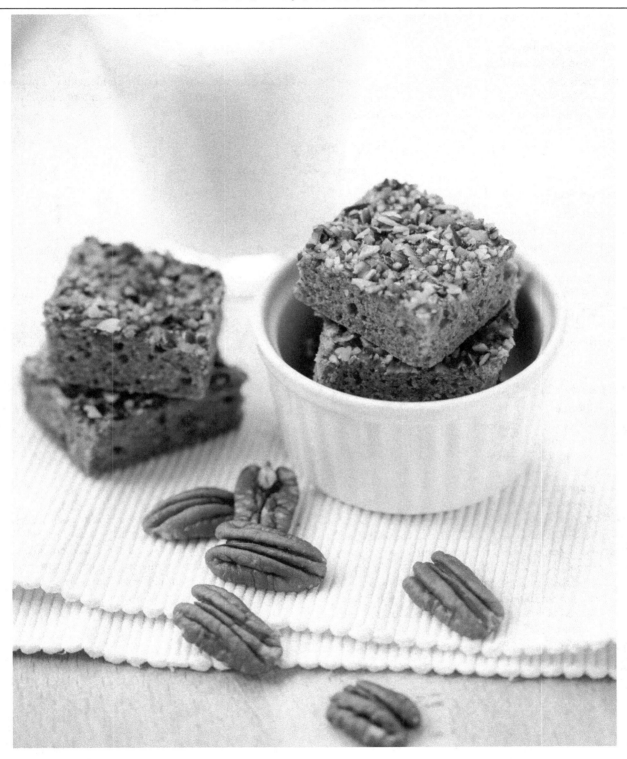

67) Chili Pepper Turnip Potatoes

Preparation Time: 50 minutes   **Servings: 4**

Ingredients:

- ✓ 4 large parsnips, sliced
- ✓ 3 tbsp ground pork rind

Directions:

- ❖ Preheat the oven to 425 F. Pour the parsnips into a bowl and add the pork rind. Stir and place parsnips on a baking sheet.

Ingredients:

- ✓ 3 tbsp olive oil
- ✓ ¼ tsp red pepper flakes
- ❖ Drizzle with olive oil and sprinkle with red pepper flakes. Bake until crispy, 40-45 minutes, tossing halfway through. Serve.

Nutrition: Calories 260; Net Carbs 22.6g; Fat 11g; Protein 3g

68) Buttery Radishes and Sauteed Steak

Preparation Time: 30 minutes   **Servings: 4**

Ingredients:

- ✓ 10 ounces tiny steak, cut into small pieces
- ✓ 3 tbsp butter
- ✓ 1½ pounds radishes, quartered

Directions:

- ❖ Melt butter in a skillet over medium heat, season meat with salt and pepper, and brown until browned on all sides, 12 minutes; transfer to a plate.

Ingredients:

- ✓ 1 clove garlic, minced
- ✓ 2 tbsp chopped fresh thyme

- ❖ Add and sauté radishes, garlic, and thyme until radishes are cooked through, 10 minutes. Plate and serve warm.

Nutrition: Calories 252; Net Carbs 0.4g; Fat 16g; Protein 21g

69) Cheddar Bacon & Celeriac Bake

Preparation Time: 50 minutes   **Servings: 4**

Ingredients:

- ✓ 6 slices bacon, chopped
- ✓ 3 tbsp butter
- ✓ 3 cloves garlic, minced
- ✓ 3 tbsp almond flour
- ✓ 2 cups coconut cream
- ✓ 1 cup chicken broth

Directions:

- ❖ Preheat oven to 400 F. Add bacon to a skillet and fry over medium heat until brown and crispy. Spoon onto a plate. Melt butter in the same skillet and sauté garlic for 1 minute. Add the almond flour and cook for another minute. Whisk in the coconut cream, chicken broth, salt and pepper. Cook on low heat for 5 minutes.

Ingredients:

- ✓ Salt and black pepper to taste
- ✓ 1 pound celeriac, peeled and sliced
- ✓ 2 cups shredded cheddar cheese
- ✓ ¼ cup chopped shallots

- ❖ Spread a layer of sauce in a greased casserole dish and arrange a layer of celeriac on top. Top with more sauce, top with some bacon and cheddar cheese, and scatter scallions on top. Repeat the layering process until all ingredients are used up. Bake for 35 minutes. Allow to rest for a few minutes and serve.

Nutrition: Calories 981; Net Carbs 20g; Fat 86g; Protein 28g

70) Chicken ham with mini peppers

Preparation Time: 30 minutes

Servings: 4

Ingredients:
- ✓ 12 mini green peppers, halved and seeded
- ✓ 4 slices chicken ham, chopped
- ✓ 1 tbsp chopped parsley
- ✓ 8 ounces cream cheese

Directions:
- ❖ Preheat oven to 400 F. Place peppers in a greased baking dish and set aside. In a bowl, combine the chicken ham, parsley, cream cheese, hot sauce and butter.

Ingredients:
- ✓ ½ tbsp hot sauce
- ✓ 2 tbsp melted butter
- ✓ 1 cup shredded gruyere cheese

- ❖ Spread the mixture into the peppers and sprinkle with Gruyere cheese. Bake until cheese melts, about 20 minutes. Serve.

Nutrition: Calories 408; Net carbohydrates 4g; Fat 32g; Protein 19g

71) Crispy Baked Asparagus with Cheese

Preparation Time: 40 minutes

Servings: 4

Ingredients:
- ✓ 1 cup grated Pecorino Romano cheese
- ✓ 4 slices Serrano ham, chopped
- ✓ 2 pounds asparagus, stalks chopped
- ✓ ¾ cup coconut cream

Directions:
- ❖ Preheat oven to 400 F. Arrange the asparagus on a greased baking sheet and pour the coconut cream over it. Scatter the garlic, serrano ham and pork rinds and sprinkle with the pecorino cheese, mozzarella cheese and paprika.

Ingredients:
- ✓ 3 cloves garlic, minced
- ✓ 1 cup crushed pork rind
- ✓ 1 cup grated mozzarella cheese
- ✓ ½ tsp sweet paprika
- ❖ Bake until cheese is melted and golden brown and asparagus is tender, 30 minutes.
- ❖ Serve warm.

Nutrition: Calories 361; Net Carbs 15g; Fat 21g; Protein 32g

72) Easy bacon and cheese balls

Preparation Time: 30 minutes

Servings: 4

Ingredients:
- ✓ 7 slices of bacon
- ✓ 6 ounces of cream cheese
- ✓ 6 ounces shredded Gruyere cheese

Directions:
- ❖ Place bacon in a skillet and fry over medium heat until crispy, 5 minutes. Transfer to a plate to cool and crisp. Pour the bacon grease into a bowl and stir in the cream cheese, Gruyere cheese, butter and red pepper flakes.

Ingredients:
- ✓ 2 tbsp softened butter
- ✓ ½ tsp red pepper flakes

- ❖ Place in the refrigerator to rest for 15 minutes. Remove and shape into walnut-sized balls. Roll in crumbled bacon. Plate and serve.

Nutrition: Calories 538; Net Carbs 0.5g; Fat 50g; Protein 22g

73) Cauliflower sauteed with bacon

Preparation Time: 15 minutes

Servings: 4

Ingredients:

- ✓ 1 large head of cauliflower, cut into florets
- ✓ 10 ounces bacon, chopped
- ✓ 1 clove garlic, minced

Directions:

- ❖ Pour cauliflower into boiling salted water over medium heat and cook for 5 minutes or until soft; drain and set aside.

Ingredients:

- ✓ Salt and black pepper to taste
- ✓ 2 tbsp parsley, finely chopped

- ❖ In a skillet, fry bacon until brown and crisp, 5 minutes. Add cauliflower and garlic and sauté until cauliflower is lightly browned. Season with salt and pepper. Garnish with parsley and serve.

Nutrition: Calories 243; Net Carbs 3.9g; Fat 21g; Protein 9g

74) Roasted mixed vegetables

Preparation Time: 40 minutes

Servings: 4

Ingredients:

- ✓ 2 lb butternut squash, cut into chunks
- ✓ ¼ lb pearl onions, peeled
- ✓ 2 rutabagas, cut into chunks
- ✓ 1 lb brussels sprouts
- ✓ Salt and black pepper to taste

Directions:

- ❖ Preheat the oven to 450°F. Pour the squash, pearl onions, rutabaga, garlic cloves, and Brussels sprouts into a bowl. Season with salt, black pepper, and olive oil and toss to combine.

Ingredients:

- ✓ 1 sprig rosemary, chopped
- ✓ 1 sprig thyme, chopped
- ✓ 4 garlic cloves, peeled only
- ✓ 3 tbsp olive oil

- ❖ Pour the mixture onto a baking sheet and sprinkle with the chopped thyme and rosemary. Roast the vegetables for 15-20 minutes. Once ready, remove and place in a serving bowl. Serve with baked chicken thighs.

Nutrition: Calories 65, fat 3g, net carbs 8g, protein 3g

75) Green bean chips with cheese

Preparation Time: 30 minutes

Servings: 6

Ingredients:

- ✓ ¼ cup Pecorino cheese, grated
- ✓ ¼ cup pork rind crumbs
- ✓ 1 tsp garlic powder

Directions:

- ❖ Preheat oven to 425°F and line a baking sheet with aluminum foil. Mix the cheese, pork rind, garlic powder, salt and black pepper in a bowl. Beat the eggs in another bowl.

Ingredients:

- ✓ Salt and black pepper to taste
- ✓ 2 eggs
- ✓ 1 pound green beans, stringless
- ❖ Dip the green beans in the eggs, then in the cheese mixture and arrange evenly on the baking sheet. Lightly grease with cooking spray and bake for 15 minutes to crisp. Transfer to a wire rack to cool before serving. Serve with a sugar-free tomato sauce.

Nutrition: Calories 210, Fat 19g, Net Carbs 3g, Protein 5g

76) Jalapeño Poppers Wrapped in Bacon

Preparation Time: 30 minutes

Servings: 6

Ingredients:
- ✓ 12 jalapeno peppers
- ✓ ¼ cup shredded Colby cheese

Ingredients:
- ✓ 6 ounces cream cheese, softened
- ✓ 6 slices of bacon, cut in half

Directions:
- ❖ Cut the jalapeno peppers in half, then remove the membrane and seeds. Combine the cheeses and stuff the bell pepper halves. Wrap each bell pepper with a strip of bacon and secure with toothpicks.

- ❖ Place the stuffed peppers on a baking sheet lined with aluminum foil. Bake at 350°F for 25 minutes until the bacon is golden brown and crispy and the cheese is golden brown on top. Remove to a paper towel-lined plate to absorb the grease, arrange on a serving platter and serve warm.

Nutrition: Calories 206, Fat 17g, Net Carbs 0g, Protein 14g

77) Garlic Cheddar Cookies

Preparation Time: 20 minutes

Servings: 4

Ingredients:
- ✓ ⅓ cup almond flour
- ✓ 2 tsp garlic powder
- ✓ Salt to taste
- ✓ 1 tsp baking powder

Ingredients:
- ✓ 5 eggs
- ✓ ⅓ cup melted butter
- ✓ 1 ¼ cups sharp cheddar cheese, grated
- ✓ ⅓ cup Greek yogurt
- ❖ Mix well until a dough-like consistency has formed. Scoop half a tbsp of batter onto a greased baking sheet with 2-inch intervals between batters. Bake for 12 minutes to golden brown. Serve cooled.

Directions:
- ❖ Preheat oven to 350°F. Mix the almond flour, garlic powder, salt, baking powder and cheddar in a bowl. In a separate bowl, beat the eggs, butter and Greek yogurt and then pour them into the dry ingredients.

Nutrition: Calories 153, Fat 14.2g, Net Carbs 1.4g, Protein 5.4g

78) Herb cheese sticks

Preparation Time: 15 minutes

Servings: 4

Ingredients:
- ✓ 1 cup pork rind, crushed
- ✓ 1 tbsp Italian herb blend

Ingredients:
- ✓ 1 egg
- ✓ 1 pound Swiss cheese, cut into sticks
- ❖ Then, generously dip in the pork rind mixture. Arrange on the baking sheet. Bake for 4 to 5 minutes, remove later, let cool for 2 minutes and serve with marinara sauce.

Directions:
- ❖ Preheat oven to 350°F. Line a baking sheet with parchment paper. Combine the pork rind and herb mix in a bowl to be evenly mixed and beat the egg in another bowl. Coat the cheese sticks in the egg.

Nutrition: Calories 188, Fat 17.3g, Net Carbs 0g, Protein 8g

79) Mozzarella and Prosciutto Bands

Preparation Time: 15 minutes

Servings: 6

Ingredients:
- ✓ 6 thin slices of prosciutto
- ✓ 18 basil leaves

Directions:
- ❖ Cut the prosciutto slices into three strips each. Place the basil leaves at the end of each strip. Add a scoop of cherry mozzarella.

Ingredients:
- ✓ 18 mozzarella cherry balls
- ✓ 2 tbsp of extra virgin olive oil
- ❖ Wrap the mozzarella in the prosciutto. Secure with toothpicks. Arrange on a serving platter, drizzle with olive oil and serve.

Nutrition: Calories 163, Fat: 12g, Net Carbohydrates: 0.1g, Protein: 13g

80) Avocado and Walnut Croutons

Preparation Time: 15 minutes

Servings: 4

Ingredients:
- ✓ 8 slices of zero carb bread
- ✓ 4 sheets of nori
- ✓ 1 avocado, pitted and chopped
- ✓ ⅓ tsp salt

Directions:
- ❖ In a bowl, mash the avocado with a fork. Add the salt and lemon juice and toss to combine. Place the bread slices on a baking sheet and toast them under the broiler for 3-4 minutes until golden brown.

Ingredients:
- ✓ 1 tsp lemon juice
- ✓ 1 ½ tbsp coconut oil
- ✓ ⅓ cup walnuts, chopped
- ✓ 1 tbsp poppy seeds
- ❖ Remove them and brush them with the coconut oil and spread the avocado puree on top. Garnish with the poppy seeds and walnuts, serve.

Nutrition: Calories 195, Fat 12.2g, Net Carbs 2.8g, Protein 13.7g

81) Parmesan Biscuits

Preparation Time: 25 minutes

Servings: 6

Ingredients:
- ✓ 1 ⅓ cups coconut flour
- ✓ 1 ¼ cups grated Parmesan cheese
- ✓ Salt and black pepper to taste
- ✓ 1 tsp garlic powder

Directions:
- ❖ Preheat oven to 350°F. Mix the coconut flour, Parmesan cheese, salt, pepper, garlic powder and paprika in a bowl. Add the butter and mix well. Add the heavy cream and mix again until a smooth, thick mixture forms. Add 1 to 2 tbsp of water at this point if it is too thick.

Ingredients:
- ✓ ⅓ cup butter, softened
- ✓ ⅓ tsp sweet paprika
- ✓ ⅓ cup heavy cream
- ✓ ⅓ tsp cumin seeds
- ❖ Place the dough on a cutting board and cover with plastic wrap. Use a rolling pin to roll out the dough into a light rectangle. Cut cookie squares from the dough and place them on a baking sheet without overlapping. Sprinkle with cumin seeds. Bake for 20 minutes. Serve chilled.

Nutrition: Calories 115, Fat 3g, Net Carbs 0.7g, Protein 5g

82) Spiced stuffed eggs with herbs

Preparation Time: 30 minutes

Servings: 4

Ingredients:
- ✓ 12 large eggs
- ✓ 6 tbsp of mayonnaise
- ✓ Salt and pepper to taste
- ✓ 1 tsp mixed dried herbs
- ✓ ½ tsp Worcestershire sauce

Ingredients:
- ✓ ¼ tsp Dijon mustard
- ✓ ½ tsp sweet paprika
- ✓ 2 tbsp fresh parsley, chopped

Directions:
- ❖ Pour salted water into a saucepan and bring to a boil over high heat. Add eggs and cook for 10 minutes. Remove to an ice bath and allow to cool. Peel and cut in half lengthwise and place yolks in a bowl.

- ❖ Use a fork to mash them. Add the mayonnaise, salt, chili, dried herbs, Worcestershire sauce, mustard and paprika. Mix until a smooth paste forms. Then, pour the mixture into a pastry bag and fill in the egg white holes. Garnish with parsley and serve immediately.

Nutrition: Calories 112, Fat 9.3g, Net Carbs 0.4g, Protein 6.7g

83) Roast green beans and mozzarella cheese with bacon

Preparation Time: 30 minutes

Servings: 4

Ingredients:
- ✓ 2 tbsp olive oil
- ✓ 1 tsp of onion powder
- ✓ 1 beaten egg

Ingredients:
- ✓ 15 ounces fresh green beans
- ✓ 5 tbsp grated mozzarella cheese
- ✓ 4 slices bacon, chopped
- ❖ Pour the mixture onto the baking sheet and bake until the green beans turn slightly brown and the cheese melts, 20 minutes. Fry the bacon in a skillet until crisp and brown. Remove green beans and divide among serving plates. Add bacon and serve.

Directions:
- ❖ Preheat oven to 350 F. Line a baking sheet with parchment paper. In a bowl, mix the olive oil, onion and garlic powder, and egg. Add the green beans and mozzarella cheese and stir to coat.

Nutrition: Calories 208; Net carbs 2.6g; Fat 19g; Protein 6g

84) Salami and cheese skewers

Preparation Time: 10 minutes + cooling time

Servings: 4

Ingredients:
- ✓ ¼ cup olive oil
- ✓ 1 tbsp plain vinegar
- ✓ 2 cloves garlic, minced
- ✓ 1 tsp dried Italian herb mixture

Ingredients:
- ✓ 4 ounces hard salami, cubed
- ✓ ¼ cup pitted Kalamata olives
- ✓ 12 ounces cheddar cheese, cubed
- ✓ 1 tsp chopped parsley
- ❖ Remove, drain marinade and thread a cube of salami, olive and cheese cube onto a skewer. Repeat by making more skewers with the remaining ingredients. Garnish with parsley and serve.

Directions:
- ❖ In a bowl, mix olive oil, vinegar, garlic and herb mixture. Add salami, olives and cheddar cheese. Stir until well coated. Cover bowl with plastic wrap and marinate in refrigerator for 4 hours.

Nutrition: Calories 585; Net carbs 1.8g; Fat 52g; Protein 27g

85) Baked zucchini sticks with chili and Aioli

Preparation Time: 25 minutes

Servings: 4

Ingredients:

- ✓ ¼ cup Pecorino Romano cheese, shredded
- ✓ ¼ cup pork rind crumbs
- ✓ 1 tsp sweet paprika
- ✓ Salt and chili pepper to taste
- ✓ 1 cup mayonnaise

Directions:

- ❖ Preheat oven to 425 F. Line a baking sheet with aluminum foil. In a bowl, mix the pork rinds, paprika, pecorino romano, salt and pepper. Beat the eggs in another bowl. Coat the zucchini strips in the eggs, then in the cheese mixture and arrange on the baking sheet.

Nutrition: Calories 180; Net carbs 2g; Fat 14g; Protein 6g

Ingredients:

- ✓ Juice of half a lemon
- ✓ 2 cloves of garlic, minced
- ✓ 3 fresh eggs
- ✓ 2 zucchini, cut into strips

- ❖ Lightly grease with cooking spray and bake for 15 minutes. Combine the mayonnaise, lemon juice, and garlic in a bowl and mix gently until everything is well incorporated. Serve the strips with the aioli.

86) Cauliflower rice and bacon gratin

Preparation Time: 30 minutes   **Servings: 4**

Ingredients:

- ✓ 1 cup canned artichoke hearts, drained and chopped
- ✓ 6 slices bacon, chopped
- ✓ 2 cups cauliflower rice
- ✓ 3 cups spinach, chopped
- ✓ 1 clove garlic, minced
- ✓ 1 tbsp olive oil

Directions:

- ❖ Preheat oven to 350 F. Cook bacon in a skillet over medium heat until brown and crispy, 5 minutes. Spoon onto a plate. In a bowl, mix Cauli rice, artichokes, spinach, garlic, olive oil, salt, pepper, sour cream, cream cheese, bacon and half of the Parmesan cheese.

Nutrition: Calories 500; Net Carbs 5.3g; Fat 37g; Protein 28g

Ingredients:

- ✓ Salt and black pepper to taste
- ✓ ¼ cup sour cream
- ✓ 8 ounces cream cheese, softened
- ✓ ¼ cup grated Parmesan cheese
- ✓ 1 ½ cups grated mozzarella cheese

- ❖ Spread the mixture on a baking sheet and top with the remaining Parmesan and mozzarella. Bake for 15 minutes. Serve.

87) Delicious Strawberries with Bacon

Preparation Time: 30 minutes   **Servings: 4**

Ingredients:

- ✓ 2 tbsp powdered sugar swerve
- ✓ 1 cup mascarpone cheese
- ✓ 1/8 tsp white pepper

Directions:

- ❖ In a bowl, combine the mascarpone, powdered sugar and white pepper. Coat the strawberries in the mixture, wrap each strawberry in a slice of bacon, and place on an ungreased baking sheet.

Nutrition: Calories 171; Net Carbs 1.2g; Fat 11g; Protein 12g

Ingredients:

- ✓ 12 fresh strawberries
- ✓ 12 thin slices of bacon

- ❖ Bake at 425 F for 15-20 minutes until bacon is brown. Serve warm.

88) Creamy ham and parsnip puree

Preparation Time: 45 minutes

Servings: 4

Ingredients:
- ✓ 1 pound parsnips, diced
- ✓ 3 tbsp olive oil, divided
- ✓ 2 tsp garlic powder
- ✓ ¾ cup almond milk

Ingredients:
- ✓ 4 tbsp heavy cream
- ✓ 4 tbsp butter
- ✓ 6 slices prosciutto, chopped
- ✓ 2 tsp fresh oregano, chopped

Directions:
- ❖ Preheat oven to 400 F. Spread parsnips on a baking sheet and drizzle with 2 tbsp olive oil. Cover tightly with aluminum foil and bake until the parsnips are tender, 40 minutes.

- ❖ Remove from oven, remove foil and transfer to a bowl. Add the garlic powder, almond milk, heavy cream and butter. Using an immersion blender, blend ingredients until smooth. Add the ham and sprinkle with oregano. Serve.

Nutrition: Calories 477; Net carbs 20g; Fat 30g; Protein 10g

89) Roasted ham with radishes

Preparation Time: 30 minutes

Servings: 4

Ingredients:
- ✓ 1 pound radishes, halved
- ✓ Salt and black pepper to taste

Ingredients:
- ✓ 1 tbsp melted butter
- ✓ 3 slices ham, chopped

Directions:
- ❖ Preheat oven to 375 F. Arrange radishes on a greased baking sheet.

- ❖ Season with salt and pepper and sprinkle with butter and ham. Bake for 25 minutes. Serve warm.

Nutrition: Calories 68; Net Carbs 0.5g; Fat 4g; Protein 4g

90) Rosemary cheese chips with guacamole

Preparation Time: 20 minutes

Servings: 4

Ingredients:
- ✓ 1 tbsp rosemary, chopped
- ✓ 1 cup Grana Padano cheese, grated
- ✓ ¼ tsp sweet paprika

Ingredients:
- ✓ ¼ tsp garlic powder
- ✓ 2 avocados, pitted and mashed
- ✓ 1 tomato, chopped
- ❖ To make the guacamole, mash the avocado with a fork in a bowl, add the tomato and continue mashing until smooth; season. Serve the chips with the guacamole.

Directions:
- ❖ Preheat oven to 350 F. Line a baking sheet with parchment paper. Mix Grana Padano cheese, paprika, rosemary and garlic powder evenly. Spread 6-8 tsp on baking sheet, creating spaces between each pile; flatten piles. Bake for 5 minutes, cool and remove to a plate.

Nutrition: Calories 229; Net Carbs 2g; Fat 20g; Protein 10g

91) Ham rolls with chives and green beans

Preparation Time: 15 minutes + cooling time

Servings: 4

Ingredients:
- ✓ 8 ounces Havarti cheese, cut into 16 strips
- ✓ 16 thin slices of prosciutto, cut in half lengthwise
- ✓ 1 medium sweet red bell pepper, cut into 16 strips
- ✓ 1 ½ cups water

Directions:
- ❖ Bring water to a boil in a saucepan over medium heat. Add green beans, cover and cook for 3 minutes or until softened; drain. Melt butter in a skillet and sauté green beans for 2 minutes; transfer to a plate.

Ingredients:
- ✓ 16 fresh green beans
- ✓ 2 tbsp salted butter
- ✓ 16 whole chives

- ❖ Assemble 1 green bean, 1 strip of red bell pepper, 1 strip of cheese and wrap with a slice of ham. Tie with a chive. Repeat assembly process with remaining ingredients and refrigerate.

Nutrition: Calories 399; Net carbs 8.7g; Fat 24g; Protein 35g

92) Crunchy rutabaga puff pastries

Preparation Time: 35 minutes

Servings: 4

Ingredients:
- ✓ 1 rutabaga, peeled and diced
- ✓ 2 tbsp melted butter

Directions:
- ❖ Preheat oven to 400 F. Spread the rutabaga on a baking sheet and drizzle with butter. Bake until tender, 15 minutes. Transfer to a bowl. Allow to cool and add the goat cheese. Using a fork, mash and mix ingredients together.

Ingredients:
- ✓ ½ oz goat cheese, crumbled
- ✓ ¼ cup ground pork rinds
- ❖ Pour pork rinds onto a plate. Form 1-inch balls with the rutabaga mixture and roll them properly in the pork rind, pressing gently to adhere. Place in the same baking dish and bake for 10 minutes until golden brown. Serve.

Nutrition: Calories 129; Net carbohydrates 5.9g; Fat 8g; Protein 3g

93) Crispy Roast Bacon and Butternut Squash

Preparation Time: 30 minutes

Servings: 4

Ingredients:
- ✓ 2 butternut squash, cut into cubes
- ✓ 1 tsp turmeric powder
- ✓ ½ tsp garlic powder

Directions:
- ❖ Preheat the oven to 425 F. In a bowl, add the squash, turmeric, garlic powder, bacon and olive oil. Stir until well coated.

Ingredients:
- ✓ 8 slices of bacon, chopped
- ✓ 2 tbsp olive oil
- ✓ 1 tbsp chopped cilantro,
- ❖ Spread the mixture onto a greased baking sheet and roast for 10-15 minutes. Transfer vegetables to a bowl and garnish with cilantro to serve.

Nutrition: Calories 148; Net Carbs 6.4g; Fat 10g; Protein 6g

94) Eggs with paprika and dill

Preparation Time: 20 minutes

Servings: 4

Ingredients:
- ✓ 1 tsp dill, chopped
- ✓ 8 large eggs
- ✓ 3 cups water

Directions:
- ❖ Bring eggs to a boil in salted water and cook for 10 minutes. Transfer to an ice water bath, let cool completely and peel the shells. Cut the eggs in half lengthwise and empty the yolks into a bowl. Mash with a fork and mix with the sriracha sauce, mayonnaise and paprika until smooth.

Ingredients:
- ✓ 3 tbsp sriracha sauce
- ✓ 4 tbsp mayonnaise
- ✓ ¼ tsp sweet paprika
- ❖ Pour filling into a pastry bag and fill egg whites so they are slightly above the rim. Garnish with dill and serve.

Nutrition: Calories 195; Net carbs 1g; Fat 19g; Protein 4g

95) Plain Stuffed Eggs with Mayonnaise

Preparation Time: 30 minutes

Servings: 6

Ingredients:
- ✓ 6 eggs
- ✓ 1 tbsp tabasco verde

Directions:
- ❖ Place eggs in boiling salted water and cook for 10 minutes. Remove eggs to an ice bath and allow to cool. Peel and cut in half lengthwise.

Ingredients:
- ✓ ¼ cup mayonnaise
- ✓ 2 tbsp black olives, sliced
- ❖ Scoop the yolks into a bowl and mash them with a fork. Whisk together the tabasco, mayonnaise and crushed yolks in a bowl. Pour this mixture into the egg whites. Garnish with olives and serve.

Nutrition: Calories 178; Net carbohydrates: 5g; Fat: 17g; Protein: 6g

96) Pork rind bread with cheese

Preparation Time: 30 minutes

Servings: 4

Ingredients:
- ✓ ¼ cup grated Pecorino Romano cheese
- ✓ 8 ounces of cream cheese
- ✓ 2 cups grated mozzarella cheese
- ✓ 1 tbsp baking powder

Directions:
- ❖ Preheat oven to 375 F. Line a baking sheet with baking paper. Microwave the cream cheese and mozzarella cheese for 1 minute or until melted.

Ingredients:
- ✓ 1 cup crushed pork rind
- ✓ 3 large eggs
- ✓ 1 tbsp mixed Italian herbs

- ❖ Blend baking powder, pork rind, eggs, pecorino romano cheese and Italian mixed herbs. Spread mixture into baking dish and bake for 20 minutes until lightly brown. Let cool, slice and serve.

Nutrition: Calories 437; Net Carbs 3.2g; Fat 23g; Protein 32g

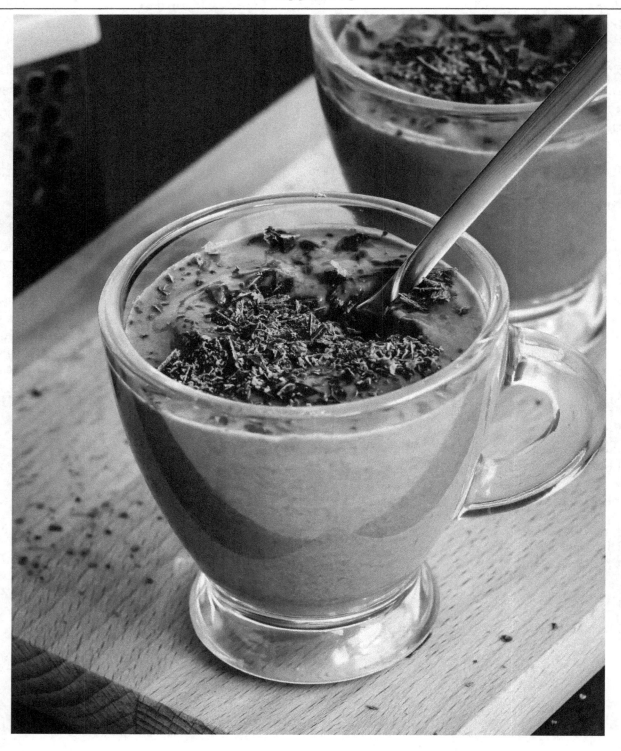

97) Orange Delight

Preparation Time: 35 minutes

Ingredients:
- ✓ Juice of 2 lemons
- ✓ 6 tbsp of stevia

Servings: 2

Ingredients:
- ✓ 1 pound of oranges, peeled and cut in half
- ✓ 1 pint of water
- ❖ Divide into jars and serve cold.

Directions:
- ❖ In Instant Pot, mix lemon juice with orange juice and orange segments, water and stevia, cover and cook over high heat for 15 minutes.

Nutrition: Calories 75 | Fat: 0g | Carbohydrates: 2g | Protein: 2g | Fiber: 0g | Sugar: 5g

98) Simple Pumpkin Pie

Preparation Time: 2 minutes

Ingredients:
- ✓ 2 pounds of pumpkin, peeled and cut into pieces
- ✓ 2 eggs
- ✓ 2 cups water
- ✓ 1 cup of coconut milk
- ✓ 2 tbsp of honey

Servings: 25

Ingredients:
- ✓ 1 tsp cinnamon powder
- ✓ ½ tsp ginger powder
- ✓ ¼ tsp. cloves, ground
- ✓ 1 tbsp arrowroot powder
- ✓ Chopped pecans
- ❖ Add the rest of the water to the Instant Pot, add the steamer basket, add ramekins inside, cover and cook on high heat for 10 minutes.
- ❖ Garnish with chopped pecans and serve.
- ❖ Enjoy!

Directions:
- ❖ Place 1 cup of water in the Instant Pot, add the steamer basket, add the pumpkin pieces, cover, cook on high heat for 4 minutes, drain, transfer to a bowl and mash.
- ❖ Add honey, milk, eggs, cinnamon, ginger and cloves, mix very well and pour into ramekins.

Nutrition: Calories 132 | Fat: 1g | Carbohydrates: 2g | Protein: 3g | Fiber: 2g | Sugar: 0g

99) Green Tea Brownies with Macadamia Nuts

Preparation Time: 28 minutes

Ingredients:
- ✓ 1 tbsp green tea powder
- ✓ ¼ cup unsalted butter, melted
- ✓ 4 tbsp powdered sugar swerve
- ✓ A pinch of salt

Servings: 4

Ingredients:
- ✓ ¼ cup coconut flour
- ✓ ½ tsp baking powder
- ✓ 1 egg
- ✓ ¼ cup chopped macadamia nuts
- ❖ Beat the mixture until the egg is incorporated. Pour the coconut flour, green tea and baking powder into a fine mesh sieve, sift into the egg bowl and stir. Add the walnuts, mix again and pour the mixture into the lined baking dish. Bake for 18 minutes, remove and dice the brownies.

Directions:
- ❖ Preheat oven to 350°F and line a square baking sheet with baking paper. Pour the melted butter into a bowl, add the sugar and salt and beat to combine. Crack the egg into the bowl.

Nutrition: Calories 248, Fat 23.1g, Net Carbs 2.2g, Protein 5.2g

100) Lychee and Coconut Lassi

Preparation Time: 30 minutes + cooling time

Servings: 4

Ingredients:
- ✓ 2 cups lychee pulp, seeded
- ✓ 2 ½ cups coconut milk
- ✓ 4 tbsp of swerve sugar
- ✓ 2 limes, peeled and squeezed

Ingredients:
- ✓ 1 ½ cups plain yogurt
- ✓ 1 lemongrass, white part only, torn off
- ✓ 2 tbsp toasted coconut flakes
- ✓ A pinch of salt
- ❖ Remove the lemongrass and pour the mixture into a smoothie machine or blender. Add the yogurt, salt, and lime juice and process the ingredients until smooth, about 60 seconds. Pour into a pitcher and refrigerate for 2 hours until cold; stir. Serve garnished with coconut shavings.

Directions:
- ❖ In a saucepan, add the lychee pulp, coconut milk, swerve sugar, lemongrass and lime zest. Stir and bring to a boil over medium heat for 2 minutes, stirring constantly. Then reduce the heat and simmer for 1 minute. Turn off the heat and let the mixture sit for 15 minutes.

Nutrition: Calories 285, Fat 26.1g, Net Carbs 1.5g, Protein 5.3g

101) Lemon Cheesecake Mousse

Preparation Time: 5 minutes + cooling time

Servings: 4

Ingredients:
- ✓ 24 ounces cream cheese, softened
- ✓ 2 cups powdered sugar swerve
- ✓ 2 lemons, squeezed and peeled

Ingredients:
- ✓ ¼ tsp salt
- ✓ 1 ¼ cups whipped cream

- ❖ Pour mousse into serving cups and refrigerate to thicken for 1 hour. Drizzle with remaining whipped cream and lightly garnish with lemon zest. Allow to rest in the refrigerator before serving.

Directions:
- ❖ Whip the cream cheese in a bowl with a hand mixer until light and fluffy. Mix in the swerve sugar, lemon juice and salt. Add 1 cup of the whipped cream to combine evenly.

Nutrition: Calories 223, fat 18g, net carbs 3g, protein 12g

102) Chocolate Mint Protein Smoothie

Preparation Time: 4 minutes

Servings: 4

Ingredients:
- ✓ 3 cups of flax milk, chilled
- ✓ 3 tbsp unsweetened cocoa powder
- ✓ 1 avocado, pitted, peeled, sliced
- ✓ 1 cup coconut milk, cooled

Ingredients:
- ✓ 3 mint leaves + more for garnish
- ✓ 3 tbsp erythritol
- ✓ 1 tbsp low-carb protein powder
- ✓ Whipping cream for garnish
- ❖ Pour into serving glasses, lightly top with whipping cream and garnish with mint leaves.

Directions:
- ❖ Combine milk, cocoa powder, avocado, coconut milk, mint leaves, erythritol and protein powder in a blender and blend for 1 minute until smooth.

Nutrition: Calories 191, Fat 14.5g, Net Carbs 4g, Protein 15g

103)   Chia and blackberry pudding

Preparation Time: 10 minutes + cooling time

Servings: 2

Ingredients:
- ✓ 1 cup whole natural yogurt
- ✓ 2 tbsp sugar swerve
- ✓ 2 tbsp chia seeds

Directions:
- ❖ In a bowl, mix the yogurt and swerve sugar. Stir in the chia seeds. Reserve 4 blackberries for garnish. Mash the remaining ones with a fork. Stir into yogurt mixture.

Ingredients:
- ✓ 1 cup fresh blackberries
- ✓ 1 tbsp lemon zest
- ✓ Mint leaves, to serve
- ❖ Refrigerate for 30 minutes. Divide the mixture between 2 glasses. Add a couple of blackberries, the mint and lemon zest to each. Serve.

Nutrition: Calories 169, Fat: 10g, Net Carbs: 4.7g, Protein: 7.5g

104)   Strawberry and Basil Lemonade

Preparation Time: 3 minutes

Servings: 4

Ingredients:
- ✓ 4 cups water
- ✓ 12 strawberries, leafless
- ✓ 1 cup fresh lemon juice
- ✓ ⅓ cup fresh basil

Directions:
- ❖ Pour crushed ice into 4 serving glasses and set aside. In a pitcher, add the water, strawberries, lemon juice, basil and swerve. Turn on the blender and process the ingredients for 30 seconds.

Ingredients:
- ✓ ¾ cup sugar swerve
- ✓ Crushed ice
- ✓ Halved strawberries for garnish
- ✓ Basil leaves for garnish
- ❖ The mixture should be pink, and the basil finely chopped. Adjust taste. Drop 2 strawberry halves and some basil into each glass and serve immediately.

Nutrition: Calories 66, Fat 0.1g, Net Carbs 5.8g, Protein 0.7g

105)   Vanilla Chocolate Mousse

Preparation Time: 30 minutes

Servings: 4

Ingredients:
- ✓ 3 eggs
- ✓ 1 cup dark chocolate chips
- ✓ 1 cup heavy cream

Directions:
- ❖ Melt the chocolate in a bowl, in your microwave for one minute on high speed, and let it cool for 10 minutes.
- ❖ Meanwhile, in a medium sized bowl, whip the cream until very smooth.

Ingredients:
- ✓ 1 cup fresh strawberries, sliced
- ✓ 1 vanilla extract
- ✓ 1 tbsp sugar swerve
- ❖ Add the eggs, vanilla extract, and reserve; beat to combine. Add the cooled chocolate. Divide the mousse among four glasses, top with the strawberry slices and chill in the refrigerator for at least 30 minutes before serving.

Nutrition: Calories 370, Fat: 25g, Net Carbs: 3.7g, Protein: 7.6g

106) Cranberry chocolate barks

Preparation Time: 5 minutes + cooling time

Servings: 6

Ingredients:
- ✓ 10 ounces unsweetened dark chocolate, chopped
- ✓ ½ cup erythritol
- ✓ ⅓ cup dried blueberries, chopped

Ingredients:
- ✓ ⅓ cup toasted walnuts, chopped
- ✓ ¼ tbsp darkened race
- ✓ ¼ tsp salt
- ❖ Stir in blueberries, dark rum, walnuts and salt, reserving some blueberries and walnuts for garnish.
- ❖ Pour the mixture onto the baking sheet and spread it out. Sprinkle with the remaining blueberries and walnuts. Refrigerate for 2 hours to rest. Break into bite-size pieces to serve.

Directions:
- ❖ Line a baking sheet with parchment paper. Pour the chocolate and erythritol into a bowl, and melt in the microwave for 25 seconds, stirring three times until completely melted.

Nutrition: Calories 225, Fat 21g, Net Carbs 3g, Protein 6g

107) Chocolate Cheesecake Bites

Preparation Time: 4 minutes + cooling time

Servings: 12

Ingredients:
- ✓ 10 ounces unsweetened dark chocolate chips
- ✓ ½ half and half

Ingredients:
- ✓ 20 ounces cream cheese, softened
- ✓ 1 tsp vanilla extract
- ❖ Stir into chocolate mixture. Spoon into silicone muffin tins and freeze for 4 hours until firm.

Directions:
- ❖ In a saucepan, melt chocolate with half and half over low heat for 1 minute. Turn off the heat. In a bowl, beat cream cheese, swerve sugar and vanilla extract with a hand mixer until smooth.

Nutrition: Calories 241, Fat 22g, Net Carbs 3.1g, Protein 5g

108) Blueberry Popsicles

Preparation Time: 5 minutes + cooling time

Servings: 6

Ingredients:
- ✓ 3 cups blueberries
- ✓ ½ tbsp lemon juice

Ingredients:
- ✓ ¼ cup of reserved sugar

- ❖ Stir in more water if too thick. Divide mixture into ice pop molds, insert stick lid and freeze 4 hours to 1 week. When ready to serve, submerge in hot water and remove pops.

Directions:
- ❖ Pour blueberries, lemon juice, sugar swerve and ¼ cup water into a blender and blend on high speed for 2 minutes until smooth. Strain through a sieve into a bowl, discarding solids.

Nutrition: Calories 48, Fat 1.2g, Net Carbohydrates 7.9g, Protein 2.3g

109) Special Vanilla Dessert

Preparation Time: 25 minutes   **Servings: 2**

Ingredients:

- ✓ 1 cup almond milk
- ✓ 4 tbsp of flax flour
- ✓ 2 tbsp of coconut flour
- ✓ 2 ½ cups water

Directions:

- ❖ In your Instant Pot, mix flax meal with flour, water, stevia, milk and espresso powder, stir, cover and cook on high heat for 10 minutes.

Ingredients:

- ✓ 2 tbsp stevia
- ✓ 1 tbsp espresso powder
- ✓ 2 tbsp vanilla extract
- ✓ Coconut cream to serve
- ❖ Add vanilla extract, mix well, set aside for 5 minutes, divide into bowls and serve with coconut cream on top.
- ❖ Enjoy!

Nutrition: Calories 182 | Fat: 2g | Carbohydrates: 3g | Protein: 4g | Fiber: 10.6g | Sugar: 1g

110) Tasty and surprising dessert with pears

It's easy to make this tasty and unique dish

Preparation Time: 25 minutes   **Servings: 2**

Ingredients:

- ✓ 1 cup water
- ✓ 2 cups of pear, peeled and diced
- ✓ 2 cups of coconut milk
- ✓ 1 tbsp of ghee
- ✓ ¼ cup brown stevia

Directions:

- ❖ In a heatproof dish, mix milk with stevia, ghee, flax meal, cinnamon, raisins, pears and walnuts and stir.
- ❖ Place water in Instant Pot, add steamer basket, place heatproof dish inside, cover and cook on high heat for 6 minutes.

Ingredients:

- ✓ ½ tbsp cinnamon powder
- ✓ 4 tbsp flax meal
- ✓ ½ cup walnuts, chopped
- ✓ ½ cup raisins

- ❖ Divide this large dessert into small cups and serve cold.
- ❖ Enjoy!

Nutrition: Calories 162 | Fat: 3g | Carbohydrates: 2g | Protein: 6g | Fiber: 1g | Sugar: 1g

111) Strawberry and Vanilla Smoothie

Preparation Time: 2 minutes   **Servings: 4**

Ingredients:

- ✓ 2 cups strawberries, cut in half
- ✓ 12 strawberries for garnish
- ✓ ½ cup unsweetened almond milk

Directions:

- ❖ Process strawberries, milk, vanilla extract, whipping cream and swerve in a large blender for 2 minutes; process in two batches if necessary.

Ingredients:

- ✓ 2/3 tsp vanilla extract
- ✓ ½ cup heavy whipping cream
- ✓ 2 tbsp sugar swerve
- ❖ Smoothie should be frosty. Pour into glasses, thread through straws, garnish with strawberry halves and serve.

Nutrition: Kcal 285, Fat 22.6g, Net Carbs 3.1g, Protein 16g

112)   Black Currant Iced Tea

Preparation Time: 10 minutes

Ingredients:

- ✓ ½ cup sugar-free blackcurrant extract
- ✓ 6 unflavored tea bags
- ✓ Sabre to taste

Directions:

- ❖ Pour ice cubes into a pitcher and refrigerate. Bring 2 cups of water to a boil in a saucepan over medium heat for 3 minutes and turn off the heat. Stir in the sugar to dissolve it and steep the tea bags in the water for 2 minutes. Remove the bags afterwards and allow the tea to cool.

Ingredients:

- ✓ Ice cubes for serving
- ✓ Lemon slices for garnish

- ❖ Stir in the black currant extract until well incorporated, remove the pitcher from the refrigerator and pour the mixture over the ice cubes. Let sit for 3 minutes to cool and after, pour the mixture into tall glasses. Add more ice cubes, place lemon slices on the rim of the glasses and serve the iced tea.

Nutrition: Kcal 22, Fat 0g, Net Carbs 5g, Protein 0g

113)   Cinnamon Turmeric Milk

Preparation Time: 7 minutes

Servings: 4

Ingredients:

- ✓ 3 cups almond milk
- ✓ ⅓ tsp cinnamon powder
- ✓ 1 cup of brewed coffee

Directions:

- ❖ In a blender, add the almond milk, cinnamon powder, coffee, turmeric and erythritol. Blend the ingredients on medium speed for 45 seconds and pour the mixture into a saucepan.

Ingredients:

- ✓ ½ tsp turmeric powder
- ✓ 1 ½ tsp erythritol
- ✓ Cinnamon sticks for garnish
- ❖ Place the saucepan over low heat and heat for 5 minutes; do not boil. Continue to shake the pan to prevent boiling. Turn off the heat and serve in mugs of milk, with a cinnamon stick in each.

Nutrition: Kcal 132, Fat 12g, Net Carbohydrates 0.3g, Protein 3.9g

114)   Almond Butter Fat Bombs

Preparation Time: 3 minutes + cooling time

Servings: 4

Ingredients:

- ✓ ½ cup almond butter
- ✓ ½ cup coconut oil

Directions:

- ❖ Melt the butter and coconut oil in the microwave for 45 seconds, stirring twice until melted and mixed properly.

Ingredients:

- ✓ 4 tbsp unsweetened cocoa powder
- ✓ ½ cup erythritol
- ❖ Stir in the cocoa powder and erythritol until fully combined. Pour into muffin molds and refrigerate for 3 hours to harden.

Nutrition: Kcal 193, Fat 18.3g, Net Carbs 2g, Protein 4g

115) Almond Milk Hot Chocolate

Preparation Time: 7 minutes

Servings: 4

Ingredients:
- ✓ 3 cups almond milk
- ✓ 4 tbsp unsweetened cocoa powder
- ✓ 2 tbsp of swerve sugar

Ingredients:
- ✓ 3 tbsp almond butter
- ✓ Finely chopped almonds for garnish

Directions:
- ❖ In a saucepan, add the almond milk, cocoa powder and swerve sugar. Stir the mixture until the sugar dissolves. Place the saucepan on low heat to heat for 5 minutes, without boiling.

- ❖ Stir the mixture occasionally. Turn off the heat and stir in the almond butter to be incorporated. Pour hot chocolate into mugs and sprinkle with chopped almonds. Serve warm.

Nutrition: Kcal 225, Fat 21.5g, Net Carbs 0.6g, Protein 4.5g

116) Raspberry Flaxseed Dessert

Preparation Time: 5 minutes

Servings: 4

Ingredients:
- ✓ 2 cups raspberries, reserving some for garnish
- ✓ 3 cups unsweetened vanilla almond milk
- ✓ 1 cup heavy cream
- ✓ ½ cup chia seeds

Ingredients:
- ✓ ½ cup flax seeds, ground
- ✓ 4 tbsp liquid stevia
- ✓ Chopped mixed nuts for garnish

Directions:
- ❖ In a medium bowl, mash raspberries with a fork until pureed. Pour in the almond milk, heavy cream, chia seeds and liquid stevia. Stir and refrigerate the pudding overnight.

- ❖ Pour pudding into serving glasses, top with raspberries, mixed nuts and serve.

Nutrition: Kcal 390, Fat 33.5g, Net Carbs 3g, Protein 13g

117) Merry Berry

Preparation Time: 6 minutes

Servings: 4

Ingredients:
- ✓ 1 cup strawberries + extra for garnish
- ✓ 1 ½ cups blackberries
- ✓ 1 cup blueberries

Ingredients:
- ✓ 2 small beets, peeled and chopped
- ✓ 2/3 cup ice cubes
- ✓ 1 lime, squeezed

Directions:
- ❖ For extra strawberries for garnish, make a single deep cut on their sides; set aside. Add blackberries, strawberries, blueberries, beets and ice cubes to smoothie maker.

- ❖ Blend ingredients on high speed until smooth and frothy, about 60 seconds. Add the lime juice and blend for 30 seconds more. Pour the drink into tall smoothie glasses, secure the reserved strawberries on the rim of each glass, stick a straw in and serve the drink immediately.

Nutrition: Kcal 83, Fat 3g, Net Carbs 8g, Protein 2.7g

118) Cinnamon Cookies

Preparation Time: 25 minutes

Servings: 4

Ingredients:
- ✓ Cookies
- ✓ 2 cups almond flour
- ✓ ½ tsp baking soda
- ✓ ¾ cup sweetener
- ✓ ½ cup butter, softened

Directions:
- ❖ Preheat oven to 350°F. Combine all cookie ingredients in a bowl. Make 16 balls with the dough and flatten them with your hands. Combine the cinnamon and erythritol.

Ingredients:
- ✓ A pinch of salt
- ✓ Coating
- ✓ 2 tbsp erythritol sweetener
- ✓ 1 tsp cinnamon

- ❖ Dip the cookies into the cinnamon mixture and place them on a lined baking sheet. Bake for 15 minutes, until crispy.

Nutrition: Kcal 134, Fat: 13g, Net Carbs: 1.5g, Protein: 3g

119) Vanilla Frappuccino

Preparation Time: 6 minutes

Servings: 4

Ingredients:
- ✓ 3 cups unsweetened vanilla almond milk, chilled Unsweetened chocolate chips for garnish
- ✓ 2 tbsp sugar swerve
- ✓ 1 ½ cups heavy cream, chilled

Directions:
- ❖ Combine almond milk, swerve sugar, heavy cream, vanilla bean and xanthan gum in blender and process on high speed for 1 minute until smooth.

Ingredients:
- ✓ 1 vanilla bean
- ✓ ¼ tsp xanthan gum

- ❖ Pour into tall shake glasses, sprinkle with chocolate chips and serve immediately.

Nutrition: Kcal 193, Fat 14g, Net Carbs 6g, Protein 15g

120) Peanut Butter Pecan Ice Cream

Preparation Time: 36 minutes + cooling time

Servings: 4

Ingredients:
- ✓ ½ cup swerve confectioners sweetener
- ✓ 2 cups heavy cream
- ✓ 1 tbsp of erythritol
- ✓ ½ cup plain peanut butter

Directions:
- ❖ Heat the heavy cream with the peanut butter, olive oil and erythritol in a small skillet over low heat without boiling for about 3 minutes. Remove from heat. In a bowl, beat egg yolks until creamy.

Ingredients:
- ✓ 1 tbsp olive oil
- ✓ 2 egg yolks
- ✓ ½ cup pecans, chopped

- ❖ Stir the eggs into the cream mixture. Continue stirring until a thick batter has formed, about 3 minutes. Pour the cream mixture into a bowl. Place in the refrigerator for 30 minutes. Stir in confectioners' sweetener.
- ❖ Pour mixture into ice cream maker and churn according to manufacturer's instructions. Stir in pecan later and spoon mixture into baking dish. Freeze for 2 hours before serving.

Nutrition: Kcal 302, Fat 32g, Net Carbs 2g, Protein 5g

121)   Coffee Fat Bombs

Preparation Time: 3 minutes + cooling time

Servings: 6

Ingredients:

- ✓ 6 tbsp prepared coffee at room temperature
- ✓ 1 ½ cups mascarpone cheese
- ✓ ½ cup melted butter

Ingredients:

- ✓ 3 tbsp unsweetened cocoa powder
- ✓ ¼ cup erythritol

- ❖ Fill muffin pans and freeze for 3 hours until firm.

Directions:

- ❖ Beat mascarpone, butter, cocoa powder, erythritol and coffee with a hand mixer until creamy and fluffy, about 1 minute.

Nutrition: Kcal 145, fat 14g, net carbs 2g, protein 4g

122)   Mixed Berry and Mascarpone Bowl

Preparation Time: 8 minutes

Servings: 4

Ingredients:

- ✓ 4 cups of Greek yogurt
- ✓ Liquid stevia to taste
- ✓ 1 ½ cups mascarpone cheese

Ingredients:

- ✓ 1 ½ cups blueberries and raspberries
- ✓ 1 cup toasted pecans

- ❖ Divide the mixture among 4 bowls, divide the berries and pecans on top of the cream. Serve the dessert immediately.

Directions:

- ❖ Mix the yogurt, stevia and mascarpone in a bowl until evenly combined.

Nutrition: Kcal 480, Fat 40g, Net Carbs 5g, Protein 20g

123)   Crazy Delicious Pudding

Preparation Time: 45 minutes

Servings: 2

Ingredients:

- ✓ 1 tangerine, sliced
- ✓ Juice of 2 tangerines
- ✓ 3 tbsp stevia
- ✓ 4 ounces of melted ghee
- ✓ ½ cup water

Ingredients:

- ✓ 2 tbsp flax meal
- ✓ ¾ cup coconut flour
- ✓ 1 tsp baking powder
- ✓ ¾ cup almonds, ground
- ✓ Olive oil cooking spray
- ❖ Add the water to the Instant Pot, place the trivet on top, add the pan, cover and cook on high heat for 35 minutes.
- ❖ Set aside to cool, slice and serve.
- ❖ Enjoy!

Directions:

- ❖ Grease a baking dish, arrange sliced tangerine on the bottom and set aside.
- ❖ In a bowl, mix ghee with stevia, flax meal, almonds, tangerine juice, flour and baking powder, stir and spread over tangerine slices.

Nutrition: Calories 200 | Fat: 2g | Carbohydrates: 3g | Protein: 4g | Fiber: 2g | Sugar: 0g

PART B– INTRODUCTION

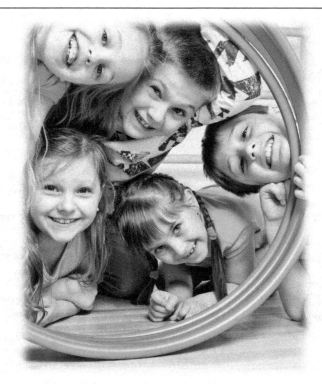

As a parent, hearing the words "diet for kids" may sound a little strange unless your child suffers from obesity. His pediatrician has recommended that he lose weight to avoid the risk of developing chronic conditions. Another possible scenario that could lead to this is if you and your partner follow the same diet or lifestyle. For example, if you are vegan, there is a high possibility that you will also raise your children as vegans. Aside from the reasons above, you may not see the essence of putting your child on a specific diet.

I can vividly recall the instance when I decided to put my children on this diet. I had been following Paleo religiously for about a year and had personally experienced the many benefits of the diet. I discovered that Paleo is one of the diets that children can follow, to my surprise and delight. It provides several health benefits for children as well.

Although food, mainly processed food, is readily available today, our early ancestors did not have access to the variety of options we have now. The foods our ancestors ate depended on their geographic conditions, the paleontological period in which they lived, and changes in the seasons. In other words, they barely had a choice - they ate only what was hunted and gathered from their environment. If they couldn't find food, they didn't eat. Despite this, our early ancestors never had to deal with as many diet-related health problems as we face today.

Nowadays, our children eat everything and whenever they want. They have gotten so used to having food at their fingertips that they barely think about the importance of eating healthy.

The Paleo diet consists of completely healthy foods like grass-fed meats, seafood, poultry, healthy oils, seeds, and nuts. With this diet, your kids will lose their uncontrollable cravings for processed and refined foods, as well as trans fats. Paleo is one of the most popular diets these days, and for a good reason. I've experienced several health benefits by sticking to this diet, such as overcoming prediabetes, brain fog, and bloating. I've also lost my excess weight! With this diet, my children and I also enjoy stable energy levels, we sleep better, our skin and hair are healthier, and we've noticed an overall improvement in our mood. Later, we'll discuss these health benefits in more detail to give you a better idea of what you and your kids should potentially expect by following this diet.

If you're a mom like me (or a dad) and you're thinking about trying Paleo, or you're already following this diet, you may also be thinking about putting your kids on Paleo. Therefore, you want to learn everything you can about Paleo for kids before you start. This is a significant first step. Educating yourself about this diet, its benefits, and how you can safely introduce it to your kids are essential steps to help you find success.

Here's another great thing about Paleo that I discovered while doing my research: according to one study, following this approach for a few days can grant you several health benefits, such as improved glucose tolerance, blood pressure, and insulin sensitivity (Frasetto et al., 2011). The same study also showed improvements in the metabolism and circulatory system of most participants.

Once you know more about Paleo, the next thing you need to think about is how to overcome the challenge of introducing this particular diet to your children. The Paleo diet is very different from the standard American diet, or the "traditional diet" that requires no rules. When introducing this diet to your children, try to think about how you would introduce a new set of rules or skills to them. Start slowly, be patient, and don't expect your children to get used to it right away. Here are some tips for getting started:

Try to find healthier alternatives for their favorite foods. This will make the transition to the Paleo diet easier.

Learn how to cook their meals and snacks, so they get used to the diet at school as well.

Add a new food to their menu every day. Avoid overwhelming your children by serving meals where everything is new. When you introduce something new, encourage them to try it.

If your children refuse to try a new type of food, avoid forcing it on them. Instead, leave it alone.

Consider involving your children in the preparation and cooking of meals. These tasks are fun, educational and can help your children learn to be more open to trying new foods.

At some point, you will need to stop preparing separate meals for your children. This is the time when you can start enjoying Paleo as a family. However, keep a side dish or dessert familiar to your children so that they still feel like they have a choice.

It is also essential that you talk about this new diet change with your children. The conversation you have with your children about Paleo depends on the age they are. Why not try a story about cave dwellers and how they ate? Then you can use it as a gateway to present your plans to start following Paleo. If you have an older child, one who already understands the concept of health, then dive right into explaining to them the benefits of this diet.

Just avoid delving into technical or scientific explanations of the benefits. Make sure your answers are age-appropriate to make sure your kids understand why you want them to start following Paleo. Communicating with your children in this way can make the whole journey much easier and positive for both parties.

As a parent interested in Paleo for kids, you will benefit immensely from this book. Here you will learn more about Paleo and what it entails. I will share tips on discussing food and nutrition with your children, how to get your family members involved in going Paleo, and how to keep this diet together. I will also share several easy and affordable recipes for you to cook in the comfort of your own home. Learning how to cook for your kids is one of the most effective ways to follow Paleo in the long run.

Since you already know your children's current diet and eating habits, learning all you can about Paleo will help you make smarter, healthier choices for them. You'll also gain valuable insights into the essential components of making any meal more Paleo-friendly and how to adjust your approach to suit your family's needs.

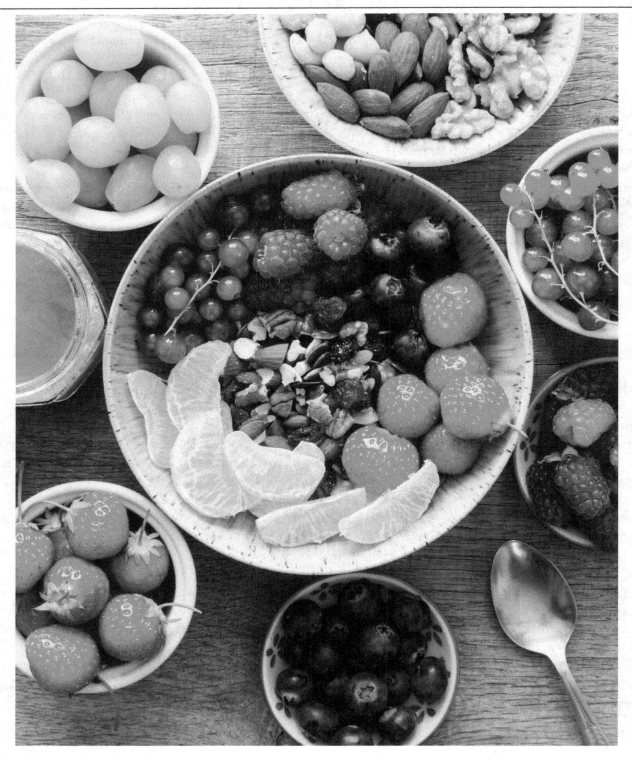

124)   Tropical Coconut Flour Bagels

Preparation Time: 25 minutes

Servings: 6

Ingredients:

- ✓ ½ cup coconut flour
- ✓ 6 eggs, beaten in a bowl
- ✓ ½ cup vegetable broth
- ✓ ¼ cup flaxseed meal

Ingredients:

- ✓ 1 tsp onion powder
- ✓ 1 tsp dried parsley
- ✓ 1 tsp chia seeds
- ✓ 1 tsp sesame seeds
- ✓ 1 onion, chopped
- ❖ Top with onion and sprinkle with chia and sesame seeds. Bake the bagels for 20 minutes. Remove and let cool before serving.

Directions:

- ❖ Preheat oven to 350°F. Mix the coconut flour, eggs, vegetable broth, flaxseed meal, onion powder, and parsley in a bowl and stir well. Spoon the mixture into a donut tray

Nutrition: Calories 426, Fat 19.1g, Net Carbs 0.4g, Protein 33.1g

125)   Spanish Chorizo and Mozzarella Omelet

Preparation Time: 15 minutes

Servings: 2

Ingredients:

- ✓ 4 eggs
- ✓ 2 oz mozzarella cheese, sliced
- ✓ 1 tbsp butter

Ingredients:

- ✓ 4 thin chorizo slices
- ✓ 1 tomato, sliced
- ✓ Salt and black pepper to taste
- ❖ Cover the skillet and cook for about 3-5 minutes until the omelet is set. Remove the pan from the heat. Run a spatula around the omelet's edges and flip it onto a plate, folded side down. Serve with salad.

Directions:

- ❖ Whisk the eggs with salt and pepper in a bowl. Melt the butter in a skillet over medium heat. Pour the eggs and cook for 1 minute. Top with the chorizo. Arrange the tomato and mozzarella over the chorizo.

Nutrition: Calories 451, Fat: 36.5g, Net Carbs: 3g, Protein: 30g

126)   Italian-style Sausage Stacks

Preparation Time: 20 minutes

Servings: 6

Ingredients:

- ✓ 6 Italian sausage patties
- ✓ 4 tbsp olive oil
- ✓ 2 ripe avocados, pitted

Ingredients:

- ✓ Salt and black pepper to taste
- ✓ 6 fresh eggs
- ✓ Red pepper flakes to garnish
- ❖ Boil 3 cups of water in a wide pan over high heat and reduce to simmer (don't boil). Crack each egg into a small bowl and gently put the egg into the simmering water. Poach for 2-3 minutes. Use a perforated spoon to remove from the water on a paper towel to dry. Repeat with the other 5 eggs. Top each stack with a poached egg and sprinkle with chili flakes. Serve with turnip wedges.

Directions:

- ❖ In a skillet, warm the oil over medium heat and fry the sausage patties about 8 minutes until lightly browned and firm. Remove the patties to a plate. Spoon the avocado into a bowl and mash it with a fork. Season with salt and black pepper. Spread the mash on the sausages.

Nutrition: Calories 378, Fat 23g, Net Carbs 5g, Protein 16g

127) Paleo Eggs and Crabmeat with Creme Fraiche Salsa

Preparation Time: 15 minutes

Servings: 3

Ingredients:

- ✓ 1 tbsp olive oil
- ✓ 6 eggs, whisked
- ✓ 1 (6 oz) can crabmeat, flaked
- ✓ Salsa
- ✓ ¾ cup crème fraiche

Directions:

- ❖ Warm the olive oil a pan over medium heat. Add in the eggs and scramble them. Stir in crabmeat and season with salt and pepper. Cook until cooked thoroughly. In a dish, combine all salsa ingredients

Ingredients:

- ✓ ½ cup scallions, chopped
- ✓ ½ tsp garlic powder
- ✓ Salt and black pepper to taste
- ✓ ½ tsp fresh dill, chopped

- ❖ . Split the egg/crabmeat mixture among serving plates. Serve alongside the scallions and salsa to the side.

Nutrition: Calories 334; Fat: 26.2g, Net Carbs: 4.4g, Protein: 21.1g

128) Easy Cheese and Aioli Eggs

Preparation Time: 20 minutes

Servings: 4

Ingredients:

- ✓ 4 eggs, hard-boiled and chopped
- ✓ 14 oz tuna in brine, drained
- ✓ ¼ lettuce head, torn into pieces
- ✓ 2 green onions, finely chopped
- ✓ ½ cup feta cheese, crumbled

Directions:

- ❖ Set the eggs in a serving bowl. Place in tuna, onion, feta cheese, lettuce, and sour cream. In a bowl, mix the mayonnaise, lemon juice, and garlic

Ingredients:

- ✓ ⅓ cup sour cream
- ✓ Aioli
- ✓ 1 cup mayonnaise
- ✓ 2 cloves garlic, minced
- ✓ 1 tbsp lemon juice
- ✓ Salt and black pepper to taste
- ❖ Season with salt and pepper. Pour the aioli into the serving bowl and stir to incorporate everything. Serve with pickles.

Nutrition: Calories 355; Fat 22.5g, Net Carbs 1.8g, Protein 29.5g

129) Special Kielbasa and Roquefort Waffles

Preparation Time: 20 minutes

Servings: 2

Ingredients:

- ✓ ½ tsp parsley, chopped
- ✓ ½ tsp chili pepper flakes
- ✓ 4 eggs

Directions:

- ❖ In a bowl, combine all ingredients except chives. Preheat the waffle iron. Pour in some batter and close the lid

Ingredients:

- ✓ ½ cup Roquefort cheese, crumbled
- ✓ 4 slices kielbasa, chopped
- ✓ 2 tbsp fresh chives, chopped
- ❖ Cook for 5 minutes until golden brown. Repeat with the rest of the batter. Decorate with chives.

Nutrition: Calories 470; Fat: 40.3g, Net Carbs: 2.9g, Protein: 24.4g

130)   Rich Baked Quail Eggs in Avocados

Preparation Time: 15 minutes

Servings: 4

Ingredients:
- ✓ 2 large avocados, halved and pitted
- ✓ 4 small eggs

Ingredients:
- ✓ Salt and black pepper to taste

Directions:
- ❖ Preheat oven to 400°F. Crack the quail eggs into the avocado halves and place them on a greased baking sheet.

- ❖ Bake the filled avocados in the oven for 8-10 minutes until eggs are cooked. Season and serve.

Nutrition: Calories 234, Fat 19.1g, Net Carbs 2.2g, Protein 8.2g

131)   Italian-style Fontina Cheese and Chorizo Waffles

Preparation Time: 30 minutes

Servings: 6

Ingredients:
- ✓ 6 eggs
- ✓ 2 tbsp butter, melted
- ✓ 1 cup almond flour

Ingredients:
- ✓ Salt and black pepper to taste
- ✓ 3 chorizo sausages, cooked, chopped
- ✓ 1 cup fontina cheese, shredded
- ❖ Preheat the waffle iron and grease it with cooking spray. Pour in the egg mixture and cook for 5 minutes until golden brown. Serve hot.

Directions:
- ❖ In a shallow bowl, beat the eggs with salt and pepper. Add in the almond milk, butter, fontina cheese, and sausages and stir to combine. Let it sit for 15-20 minutes

Nutrition: Calories 316; Fat: 25g, Net Carbs: 1.5g, Protein: 20.2g

132)   Tropical Coconut Porridge with Strawberries

Preparation Time: approx. 12 minutes

Servings: 2

Ingredients:
- ✓ Flax egg: 1 tbsp flax seed powder + 3 tbsp water
- ✓ 1 oz olive oil
- ✓ 1 tbsp coconut flour

Ingredients:
- ✓ 1 pinch ground chia seeds
- ✓ 5 tbsp coconut cream
- ✓ 1 pinch salt
- ✓ Strawberries to serve
- ❖ Cook, while stirring continuously until the desired consistency is achieved. Top with strawberries.

Directions:
- ❖ For flax egg, in a bowl, mix flax seed powder with water, and let soak for 5 minutes. Place a saucepan over low heat and pour in olive oil, flax egg, flour, chia, coconut cream, and salt.

Nutrition: Calories 521; Net Carbs 4g; Fat 49g; Protein 10g

133) Original Mexican Tofu Scramble

Preparation Time: approx. 45 minutes

Servings: 4

Ingredients:
- ✓ 8 oz tofu, scrambled
- ✓ 2 tbsp butter
- ✓ 1 green bell pepper, chopped
- ✓ 1 tomato, finely chopped

Directions:
- ❖ Melt butter in a skillet over medium heat. Fry the tofu until golden brown, stirring occasionally, about 5 minutes.

Ingredients:
- ✓ 2 tbsp chopped scallions
- ✓ Salt and black pepper to taste
- ✓ 1 tsp Mexican chili powder
- ✓ 3 oz grated Parmesan cheese
- ❖ . Stir in bell pepper, tomato, scallions, and cook until the vegetables are soft, 4 minutes. Season with salt, pepper, chili powder and stir in Parmesan cheese, about 2 minutes. Spoon the scramble into a serving platter and serve warm.

Nutrition: Calories254; Net Carbs 3g; Fat 19g; Protein 16g

134) Special No-Bread Avocado Sandwiches

Preparation Time: approx. 10 minutes

Servings: 2

Ingredients:
- ✓ 1 avocado, sliced
- ✓ 1 large red tomato, sliced
- ✓ 4 little gem lettuce leaves

Directions:
- ❖ Arrange the lettuce on a flat serving plate. Smear each leave with butter and arrange tofu slices on the leaves

Ingredients:
- ✓ ½ oz butter, softened
- ✓ 4 tofu slices
- ✓ 1 tsp chopped parsley
- ❖ Top with the avocado and tomato slices. Garnish the sandwiches with parsley and serve.

Nutrition: Calories 385; Net Carbs 4g; Fat 32g; Protein 12g

135) Easy Blueberry Chia Pudding

Preparation Time:approx. 10 min + chilling time

Servings: 2

Ingredients:
- ✓ ¾ cup coconut milk
- ✓ ½ tsp vanilla extract
- ✓ ½ cup blueberries

Directions:
- ❖ In a blender, pour coconut milk, vanilla extract, and half of the blueberries. Process the ingredients in high speed until the blueberries have incorporated into the liquid

Ingredients:
- ✓ 2 tbsp chia seeds
- ✓ 1 tbsp chopped walnuts

- ❖ . Mix in chia seeds. Share the mixture into 2 breakfast jars, cover, and refrigerate for 4 hours to allow it to gel. Garnish with the remaining blueberries and walnuts. Serve.

Nutrition: Calories 301; Net Carbs 6g; Fat 23g; Protein 9g

136)   Easy Creamy Sesame Bread

Preparation Time: approx. 40 minutes

Servings: 6

Ingredients:
- ✓ 4 tbsp flax seed powder
- ✓ 1 cup cream cheese
- ✓ 5 tbsp sesame oil
- ✓ 1 cup coconut flour

Directions:
- ❖ In a bowl, mix flax seed powder with 1 ½ cups water until smoothly combined and set aside to soak for 5 minutes. Preheat oven to 400 F. When the flax egg is ready, beat in cream cheese and 4 tbsp sesame oil until mixed. Whisk in coconut flour, psyllium husk powder, salt, and baking powder until adequately blended

Ingredients:
- ✓ 2 tbsp psyllium husk powder
- ✓ 1 tsp salt
- ✓ 1 tsp baking powder
- ✓ 1 tbsp sesame seeds
- ❖ Spread the dough in a greased baking tray. Allow to stand for 5 minutes and then brush with remaining sesame oil. Sprinkle with sesame seeds and bake the dough for 30 minutes. Slice and serve.

Nutrition: Calories 285; Net Carbs 1g; Fat 26g; Protein 8g

137)   Special Bulletproof Coffee

Preparation Time: approx. 3 minutes

Servings: 2

Ingredients:
- ✓ 2 ½ heaping tbsp ground bulletproof coffee beans
- ✓ 1 tbsp coconut oil

Directions:
- ❖ Using a coffee maker, brew one cup of coffee with the ground coffee beans and 1 cup of water. Transfer the coffee to a blender and add the coconut oil and butter

Ingredients:
- ✓ 2 tbsp unsalted butter

- ❖ Blend the mixture until frothy and smooth.

Nutrition: Calories 336; Net Carbs 0g; Fat 36g; Protein 2g

138)   Easy Breakfast Naan Bread

Preparation Time: approx. 25 minutes

Servings: 6

Ingredients:
- ✓ ¾ cup almond flour
- ✓ 2 tbsp psyllium husk powder
- ✓ 1 tsp salt
- ✓ ½ tsp baking powder

Directions:
- ❖ In a bowl, mix almond flour, psyllium husk powder, ½ tsp of salt, and baking powder. Mix in olive oil and boiling water to combine the ingredients like a thick porridge. Stir and allow the dough rise for 5 minutes. Divide the dough into 6 pieces and mold into balls. Place the balls on a parchment paper and flatten

Ingredients:
- ✓ ¼ cup olive oil
- ✓ 2 cups boiling water
- ✓ 8 oz butter
- ✓ 2 garlic cloves, minced
- ❖ . Melt half of the butter in a frying pan over medium heat and fry the naan on both sides to have a golden color. Transfer to a plate and keep warm. Add the remaining butter to the pan and sauté garlic until fragrant, about 1 minute. Pour the garlic butter into a bowl and serve as a dip along with the naan.

Nutrition: Calories 224; Net Carbs 3g; Fat 19g; Protein 4g

139) Italian Mascarpone Snapped Amaretti Biscuits

Preparation Time: 25 minutes

Servings: 6

Ingredients:

- ✓ 6 egg whites
- ✓ 1 egg yolk, beaten
- ✓ 1 tsp vanilla bean paste
- ✓ 4 tbsp swerve sugar
- ✓ A pinch of salt
- ✓ ¼ cup ground fragrant almonds

Directions:

- ❖ Preheat oven to 300°F. Line a baking sheet with parchment paper. In a bowl, beat egg whites, salt, and vanilla paste with a hand mixer while you gradually spoon in the swerve sugar until stiff. Add in almonds and fold in the egg yolk, lemon juice, and amaretto liquor. Spoon mixture into a piping bag.
- ❖ Press out 50 mounds on the baking sheet. Bake the biscuits for 15 minutes until golden brown.

Ingredients:

- ✓ 1 lemon juice
- ✓ 7 tbsp sugar-free amaretto liquor
- ✓ ¼ cup mascarpone cheese
- ✓ ¼ cup butter, room temperature
- ✓ ¾ cup swerve confectioner's sugar

- ❖ Transfer to a wire rack to cool. Whisk the mascarpone cheese, butter, and swerve confectioner's sugar with the cleaned electric mixer. Spread a scoop of mascarpone cream onto the case of half of the biscuits and snap with the remaining biscuits. Dust with some swerve confectioner's sugar and serve.

Nutrition: Calories 165, Fat 13g, Net Carbs 3g, Protein 9g

140) Special Turkey Sausage Egg Cups

Preparation Time: 15 minutes

Servings: 4

Ingredients:

- ✓ 2 tsp butter
- ✓ 8 eggs, beaten
- ✓ Salt and black pepper to taste

Directions:

- ❖ Preheat oven to 400°F. Melt butter in a skillet over medium heat. Cook the turkey sausages for 4-5 minutes. In a bowl, mix 4 eggs, sausages, cheese, and seasonings.

Ingredients:

- ✓ ½ tsp dried rosemary
- ✓ 1 cup pecorino romano, grated
- ✓ 4 turkey sausages, chopped
- ❖ Divide between greased muffin cups and bake for 4 minutes. Crack an egg into the middle of each cup. Bake for 4 more minutes. Serve cooled.

Nutrition: Calories 423; Fat: 34.1g, Net Carbs: 2.2g, Protein: 26.5g

141) Easy Cheese Stuffed Avocados

Preparation Time: 20 minutes

Servings: 4

Ingredients:

- ✓ 3 avocados, halved, pitted, skin on
- ✓ ½ cup feta cheese, crumbled
- ✓ ½ cup cheddar cheese, grated

Directions:

- ❖ Preheat oven to 360°F. Lay avocado halves in a baking dish. In a bowl, mix both types of cheeses, pepper, eggs, and salt

Ingredients:

- ✓ 2 eggs, beaten
- ✓ Salt and black pepper to taste
- ✓ 1 tbsp fresh basil, chopped
- ❖ Split the mixture into the avocado halves. Bake for 15 minutes. Top with basil and serve.

Nutrition: Calories 342; Fat: 30.4g, Net Carbs: 7.5g, Protein: 11.1g

142)   Special Duo-Cheese Omelet with Pimenta and Basil

Preparation Time: 15 minutes

Servings: 2

Ingredients:

- ✓ 1 tbsp olive oil
- ✓ 4 eggs, beaten
- ✓ Salt and black pepper to taste
- ✓ ¼ tsp paprika

Directions:

- ❖ Warm the olive oil in a pan over medium. Season the eggs with cayenne pepper, salt, paprika, and pepper. Transfer to the pan and ensure they are evenly spread. Cook for 5 minutes

Ingredients:

- ✓ ¼ tsp cayenne pepper
- ✓ ½ cup asiago cheese, shredded
- ✓ ½ cup cheddar cheese, shredded
- ✓ 2 tbsp fresh basil, roughly chopped
- ❖ Top with the asiago and cheddar cheeses. Slice the omelet into two halves. Decorate with fresh basil and serve.

Nutrition: Calories 490; Fat: 44.6g, Net Carbs: 4.5g, Protein: 22.7g

143)   Easy and Quick Blue Cheese Omelet

Preparation Time: 15 minutes

Servings: 2

Ingredients:

- ✓ 4 eggs
- ✓ Salt to taste
- ✓ 1 tbsp sesame oil

Directions:

- ❖ In a bowl, beat the eggs with salt. Warm the oil in a pan over medium heat. Add in the eggs and cook as you swirl the eggs around the pan.

Ingredients:

- ✓ ½ cup blue cheese, crumbled
- ✓ 1 tomato, thinly sliced

- ❖ Cook eggs until set. Top with cheese. Decorate with tomato and serve.

Nutrition: Calories 307Calories; Fat: 25g, Net Carbs: 2.5g, Protein: 18.5g

144)   Tropical Coconut and Walnut Chia Pudding

Preparation Time: 10 minutes

Servings: 1

Ingredients:

- ✓ ½ tsp vanilla extract
- ✓ ½ cup water
- ✓ 1 tbsp chia seeds
- ✓ 2 tbsp hemp seeds
- ✓ 1 tbsp flaxseed meal

Directions:

- ❖ Put chia seeds, hemp seeds, flaxseed meal, almond meal, stevia, and coconut in a saucepan and pour over the water. Simmer over medium heat, occasionally stirring until creamed and thickened, about 3-4 minutes

Ingredients:

- ✓ 2 tbsp almond meal
- ✓ 2 tbsp shredded coconut
- ✓ ¼ tsp granulated stevia
- ✓ 1 tbsp walnuts, chopped

- ❖ Stir in vanilla. When it is ready, spoon into a serving bowl, sprinkle with walnuts, and serve.

Nutrition: Calories Calories 334, Fat: 29g, Net Carbs: 1.5g Protein: 15g

145)   Italian Cheese Ciabatta with Pepperoni

Preparation Time: 30 minutes

Servings: 6

Ingredients:

- ✓ 10 oz cream cheese, melted
- ✓ 2 ½ cups mozzarella, shredded
- ✓ 4 large eggs, beaten
- ✓ 3 tbsp Romano cheese, grated

Directions:

- ❖ In a bowl, combine eggs, mozzarella cheese, cream cheese, baking powder, pork rinds, and Romano cheese. Form into 6 chiabatta shapes

Ingredients:

- ✓ ½ cup pork rinds, crushed
- ✓ 2 tsp baking powder
- ✓ ½ cup tomato puree
- ✓ 12 pepperoni slices
- ❖ Set a pan over medium heat. Cook each ciabatta for 2 minutes per side. Sprinkle tomato puree over each one and top with pepperoni slices to serve.

Nutrition: Calories Calories 464, Fat: 33.6g, Net Carbs: 9.1g, Protein: 31.1g

146)   Special Seed Breakfast Loaf

Preparation Time: approx. 55 minutes

Servings: 6

Ingredients:

- ✓ ¾ cup coconut flour
- ✓ 1 cup almond flour
- ✓ 3 tbsp baking powder
- ✓ 2 tbsp psyllium husk powder
- ✓ 2 tbsp desiccated coconut
- ✓ 5 tbsp sesame seeds
- ✓ ¼ cup flaxseed
- ✓ ¼ cup hemp seeds

Directions:

- ❖ Preheat oven to 350 F. In a bowl, mix coconut and almond flours, baking powder, psyllium husk, desiccated coconut, sesame seeds, flaxseed, hemp seeds, ground caraway and poppy seeds, salt, and allspice

Ingredients:

- ✓ 1 tsp ground caraway seeds
- ✓ 1 tbsp poppy seeds
- ✓ 1 tsp salt
- ✓ 1 tsp allspice
- ✓ 6 eggs
- ✓ 1 cup cream cheese, softened
- ✓ ¾ cup heavy cream
- ✓ 4 tbsp sesame oil
- ❖ In another bowl, whisk eggs, cream cheese, heavy cream, and sesame oil. Pour the mixture into the dry ingredients and combine both into a smooth dough. Pour the dough in a greased loaf pan. Bake for 45 minutes. Remove onto a rack and let cool.

Nutrition: Calories 584; Net Carbs 7.4g; Fat 50g; Protein 23g

147) Everyday Blackberry Chia Pudding

Preparation Time: approx. 45 minutes

Servings: 4

Ingredients:

- ✓ 1 ½ cups coconut milk
- ✓ ½ cup Greek yogurt
- ✓ 4 tsp sugar-free maple syrup
- ✓ 1 tsp vanilla extract
- ✓ 7 tbsp chia seeds

Ingredients:

- ✓ 1 cup fresh blackberries
- ✓ 3 tbsp chopped almonds
- ✓ Mint leaves to garnish

Directions:

- ❖ In a bowl, combine coconut milk, Greek yogurt, sugar-free maple syrup, and vanilla extract until evenly combined. Mix in the chia seeds. Puree half of blackberries in a bowl using a fork and stir in the yogurt mixture

- ❖ . Share the mixture into medium mason jars, cover the lids and refrigerate for 30 minutes to thicken the pudding. Remove the jars, take off the lid, and stir the mixture. Garnish with remaining blackberries, almonds, and some mint leaves.

Nutrition: Calories 309; Net Carbs 6.8g; Fat 26g; Protein 7g

148) Easy Blueberry Soufflé

Preparation Time: approx. 35 minutes

Servings: 4

Ingredients:

- ✓ 1 cup frozen blueberries
- ✓ 5 tbsp erythritol
- ✓ 4 egg yolks

Ingredients:

- ✓ 3 egg whites
- ✓ 1 tsp olive oil
- ✓ ½ lemon, zested
- ❖ Fold egg white mixture into egg yolk mix. Heat olive oil in a pan over low heat. Add in olive oil and pour in the egg mixture; swirl to spread. Cook for 3 minutes and transfer to the oven; bake for 2-3 minutes or until puffed and set. Plate soufflé and spoon blueberry sauce all over. Garnish with lemon zest.

Directions:

- ❖ Pour blueberries, 2 tbsp erythritol and 1 tbsp water in a saucepan. Cook until the berries soften and become syrupy, 8-10 minutes. Set aside. Preheat oven to 350 F. In a bowl, beat egg yolks and 1 tbsp of erythritol until thick and pale. In another bowl, whisk egg whites until foamy. Add in remaining erythritol and whisk until soft peak forms, 3-4 minutes.

Nutrition: Calories 99; Net Carbs 2.8g; Fat 5.9g; Protein 5.5g

149) American Cheddar Biscuits

Preparation Time: approx. 30 minutes

Servings: 4

Ingredients:

- ✓ 2 ½ cups almond flour
- ✓ 2 tsp baking powder
- ✓ 2 eggs beaten

Ingredients:

- ✓ 3 tbsp melted butter
- ✓ ¾ cup grated cheddar cheese

- ❖ Mold 12 balls out of the mixture and arrange on the sheet at 2-inch intervals. Bake for 25 minutes until golden brown. Remove, let cool, and serve.

Directions:

- ❖ Preheat oven to 350 F. Line a baking sheet with parchment paper. In a bowl, mix flour, baking powder, and eggs until smooth. Whisk in the melted butter and cheddar cheese until well combined.

Nutrition: Calories 355; Net Carbs 1.4g; Fat 28g, Protein 21g

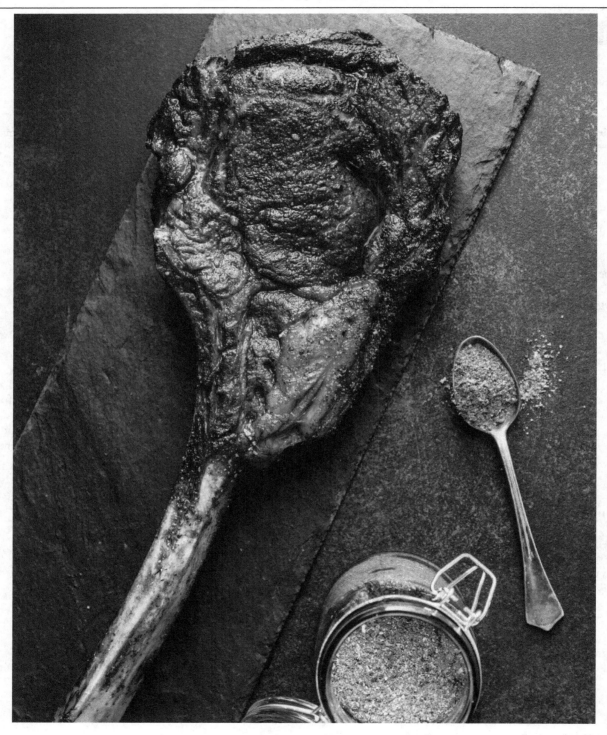

150)   Easy Paleo Shrimp Burgers

Preparation Time: 30 minutes

Servings: 4

Ingredients:

- ✓ 2 tbsp. cilantro, chopped
- ✓ 1 and ½ pounds shrimp, peeled and deveined
- ✓ 2 tbsp. chives, chopped
- ✓ Salt and pepper to aste
- ✓ 1 garlic clove, minced
- ✓ ¼ cup radishes, minced
- ✓ 1 tsp. lemon zest
- ✓ ¼ cup celery, minced
- ✓ 1 egg, whisked
- ✓ 1 tbsp. lemon juice

Ingredients:

- ✓ ¼ cup almond meal
- ✓ For the salsa:
- ✓ · 1 avocado, pitted, peeled and chopped
- ✓ · 1 cup pineapple, chopped
- ✓ · 2 tbsp. red onion, chopped
- ✓ · ¼ cup bell peppers, chopped
- ✓ · 1 tbsp. lime juice
- ✓ · 1 tbsp. cilantro, finely chopped
- ✓ · Salt and black pepper to taste

Directions:

- ❖ In a bowl, mix pineapple with avocado, bell peppers, two tbsp red onion, one tbsp lime juice, salt, pepper to the taste and one tbsp cilantro, stir well and keep in the fridge for now.
- ❖ In your food processor, mix shrimp with two tbsp cilantro, chives, and garlic and blend well.
- ❖ Transfer to a bowl and mix with radishes, celery, lemon zest, lemon juice, egg, almond meal, salt, and pepper to the taste and stir well.

- ❖ Shape 4 burgers, place them on preheated grill over medium-high heat and cook for 5 minutes on each side.
- ❖ Divide shrimp burgers between plates and serve with the salsa you've made earlier on the side.
- ❖ Enjoy!

Nutrition: Calories 238 | Fat: 12g | Carbs: 13g | Protein: 15g | Fiber: 3g | Sugar: 0g

151)   Lovely Paleo Scallops Tartar

Preparation Time: 15 minutes

Servings: 2

Ingredients:

- ✓ 6 scallops, diced
- ✓ Salt and pepper to taste
- ✓ 3 strawberries, chopped
- ✓ 1 tbsp. extra virgin olive oil

Ingredients:

- ✓ 1 tbsp. green onions, minced
- ✓ Juice of ½ lemon
- ✓ ½ tbsp. basil leaves, finely chopped

Directions:

- ❖ In a bowl, mix strawberries with scallops, basil, and onions and stir well.
- ❖ Add olive oil, salt, pepper to the taste and lemon juice and stir well again.

- ❖ Keep in the fridge until you serve.
- ❖ Enjoy!

Nutrition: Calories 180 | Fat: 27g | Carbs: 3g | Protein: 24g | Fiber: 0g | Sugar: 0g

152) Tasty Paleo Shrimp Skewers

Preparation Time: 20 minutes   **Servings: 4**

Ingredients:

- ½ lb. sausages, chopped and already cooked
- ½ lb. shrimp, peeled and deveined
- 2 tbsp. extra virgin olive oil
- 2 zucchinis, cubed
- Salt and black pepper to taste
- For the Creole seasoning:

Directions:

- ❖ In a bowl, mix paprika with garlic powder, onion one, chili powder, oregano, and thyme and stir well.
- ❖ In another bowl, combine shrimp with sausage, zucchini, and oil and toss to coat.
- ❖ Pour paprika mix over shrimp mix and stir well.

Ingredients:

- ½ tbsp. garlic powder
- 2 tbsp. paprika
- ½ tbsp. onion powder
- ¼ tbsp. oregano, dried
- ½ tbsp. chili powder
- ¼ tbsp. thyme, dried
- ❖ Arrange sausage, shrimp, and zucchini on skewers alternating pieces, place them on preheated grill over medium-high heat and cook for 8 minutes, flipping skewers from time to time.
- ❖ Arrange on a platter and serve.
- ❖ Enjoy!

Nutrition: Calories 360 | Fat: 0.8g | Carbs: 4.3g | Protein: 18.1g | Fiber: 0.8g | Sugar: 0g

153) Best Paleo Beef Stew

It's a delightful stew! The meat is so tender and succulent! It's divine!

Preparation Time: 30 minutes   **Servings: 4**

Ingredients:

- 2 lb. beef fillet, cubed
- 1 red chili, seeded and chopped
- 1 brown onion, finely chopped
- 1 tsp. ghee
- 2 tbsp. extra virgin olive oil
- Salt and black pepper to taste
- ⅔ tsp. nutmeg
- 2 tbsp. Worcestershire sauce, gluten free
- 1 garlic clove, minced
- ½ cup dried mushrooms
- ½ cup white wine
- ½ tbsp. dry sherry

Directions:

- ❖ Heat up a pot with the ghee and the olive oil over medium-high heat, add onion, chili, some salt, and pepper, stir and cook for 2-3 minutes.
- ❖ Add meat, stir and brown it for 5 minutes.
- ❖ Add Worcestershire sauce, wine, sherry, dried mushrooms, garlic, stock, thyme, fennel, rosemary, nutmeg, and star anise, stir, bring to a boil, cover, reduce heat to low and cook for 1 hour and 10 minutes.

Ingredients:

- 1 tsp. rosemary, dry
- 4 thyme springs
- ¼ tsp. fennel seeds
- 1 star anise
- 2 celery stick, chopped
- 2 carrots, thinly sliced
- 1 quart beef stock
- 6 button mushrooms, chopped
- 2 tbsp. arrowroot flour
- 1 sweet potato, chopped
- 1 tbsp. butter

- ❖ Add celery, carrots, fresh mushrooms, potato, stir, cover and cook for 15 min.
- ❖ Increase heat to medium, uncover the pot and cook the stew for 15 min.
- ❖ In a bowl, mix arrowroot flour with a cup of liquid from the stew, stir well and pour over stew.
- ❖ Also, add butter, stir well and cook for 15 more minutes.
- ❖ Transfer to bowls and serve hot.
- ❖ Enjoy!

Nutrition: Calories 113 | Fat: 8g | Carbs: 21g | Protein: 38g | Fiber: 3g | Sugar: 7g

154)   Delicious Paleo Slow Cooker Stew

Preparation Time: 2 hours

Servings:

Ingredients:

- ✓ 2 lb. beef stew meat, cubed
- ✓ 3 cups dark beer
- ✓ 7 garlic cloves, finely minced
- ✓ Salt and black pepper to taste
- ✓ 4 carrots, chopped
- ✓ 1 cup tapioca flour

Directions:

- ❖ In a bowl, mix beef with beer and three garlic cloves, toss to coat and keep in the fridge for one day.
- ❖ In a bowl, combine tapioca flour with salt and pepper to the taste and stir.
- ❖ Drain meat and reserve the 2 cups of the marinade.
- ❖ Add meat to tapioca bowls and toss to coat.
- ❖ Heat up a pan over medium-high heat, add chicken, stir and brown it for 2-3 minutes.

Ingredients:

- ✓ 2 yellow onions, finely chopped
- ✓ ½ head cabbage, finely chopped
- ✓ 30 oz. canned tomatoes, diced
- ✓ 5 yellow potatoes, chopped
- ✓ 2 cups reserved beef marinade
- ✓ 3 cups beef stock
- ❖ Transfer meat to your slow cooker.
- ❖ Add reserved marinade, carrots, cabbage, onions, tomatoes, four garlic cloves, potatoes, beef stock, salt and pepper to the taste, cover pan and cook stew on Low for 8 hours.
- ❖ Uncover pot, transfer stew to bowls and serve.
- ❖ Enjoy!

Nutrition: Calories 247 | Fat: 4.5g | Carbs: 25g | Protein: 24.2g | Fiber: 4.2g | Sugar: 1g

155)   Super Paleo Veggie and Chorizo Stew

Preparation Time: 30 minutes

Servings: 4

Ingredients:

- ✓ 1 yellow onion, chopped
- ✓ 1 tbsp. coconut oil
- ✓ 2 chorizo sausages, skinless and thinly sliced
- ✓ 1 red bell pepper, chopped
- ✓ 1 carrot, thinly sliced
- ✓ 2 white potatoes, chopped
- ✓ 1 celery stick, chopped

Directions:

- ❖ Heat up a pan with the oil over medium-high heat, add chorizo, onion, celery and carrot, stir and cook for 3 minutes.
- ❖ Add red bell pepper, tomatoes, garlic, and potato, stir and cook 1 minute.
- ❖ Add lemon juice, stock, salt, and pepper, stir, bring to a boil, cover pan, reduce heat to medium and cook for 10 minutes.

Ingredients:

- ✓ 1 tomato, chopped
- ✓ 2 garlic cloves, finely minced
- ✓ 2 cups chicken broth
- ✓ 1 tbsp. lemon juice
- ✓ Salt and black pepper to taste
- ✓ 1 zucchini, cut
- ✓ A handful parsley leaves, finely chopped
- ❖ Add zucchini, stir, cover again and cook for ten more minutes.
- ❖ Uncover pan, cook the stew for 2 minutes more stirring often.
- ❖ Add parsley, stir, take off heat, transfer to dishes and serve.
- ❖ Enjoy!

Nutrition: Calories 420 | Fat: 12g | Carbs: 45g | Protein: 33.2g | Fiber: 11g | Sugar: 0g

156) Delicious Beef and Plantain Stew

Preparation Time: 1 hour

Servings: 4

Ingredients:

- ✓ 6 plantains, skinless and cubed
- ✓ 2 lb. beef meat, cubed
- ✓ 3 cups collard greens, chopped
- ✓ Salt and black pepper to taste
- ✓ 3 cups water

Ingredients:

- ✓ ½ cup sweet paprika
- ✓ 3 tbsp. allspice
- ✓ ¼ cup garlic powder
- ✓ 1 tsp. chili powder
- ✓ 1 tsp. cayenne pepper
- ❖ Uncover slow cooker, leave stew to cool down for a few minutes, transfer to bowls and serve.
- ❖ Enjoy!

Directions:

- ❖ In your slow cooker, mix beef with plantains, collard greens, water, paprika, garlic powder, allspice, chili powder, cayenne, salt and pepper to the taste.
- ❖ Stir, cover pot and cook on High for 5 hours.

Nutrition: Calories 410 | Fat: 11g | Carbs: 39g | Protein: 34g | Fiber: 10g | Sugar: 0g

157) Healthy Paleo Chicken Stew

Preparation Time: 2 hours

Servings: 6

Ingredients:

- ✓ 5 garlic cloves, finely chopped
- ✓ 2 celery stalks, chopped
- ✓ 2 yellow onions, chopped
- ✓ 2 carrots, chopped
- ✓ 2 potatoes, cubed
- ✓ 30 oz. canned pumpkin puree

Ingredients:

- ✓ 2 quarts chicken stock
- ✓ 2 cups chicken meat, chopped
- ✓ ¼ cup tapioca flour
- ✓ Salt and black pepper to taste
- ✓ ½ lb. baby spinach
- ✓ ¼ tsp. cayenne pepper
- ❖ Transfer to bowls and serve hot.
- ❖ Enjoy!

Directions:

- ❖ In your slow cooker, mix chicken meat with onions, carrots, celery, potatoes, garlic, pumpkin puree, chicken stock, salt, pepper, tapioca flour and cayenne, stir well, cover and cook on low for 7 hours and 50 minutes.
- ❖ Uncover slow cooker, add spinach, cover again and cook for ten more minutes.

Nutrition: Calories 244 | Fat: 2g | Carbs: 38g | Protein: 20g | Fiber: 6g | Sugar: 0g

158) Special White Wine Salmon Shirataki Fettucine

Preparation Time: approx. 35 minutes

Servings: 4

Ingredients:

✓ 2 (8 oz) packs shirataki fettuccine
✓ 5 tbsp butter
✓ 4 salmon fillets, cubed
✓ Salt and black pepper to taste
✓ 3 garlic cloves, minced

Directions:

❖ Boil 2 cups of water in a pot. Strain the shirataki pasta t and rinse well under hot running water. Allow proper draining and pour the shirataki pasta into the boiling water. Cook for 3 minutes and strain again. Place a dry skillet and stir-fry the shirataki pasta until visibly dry, 1-2 minutes; set aside. Melt half of the butter in a skillet over medium heat; season the salmon with salt and pepper and cook for 8 minutes; set aside.

Ingredients:

✓ 1 ¼ cups heavy cream
✓ ½ cup dry white wine
✓ 1 tsp lemon zest
✓ 1 cup baby spinach

❖ Melt remaining butter to the skillet and stir in garlic. Cook for 30 seconds. Mix in heavy cream, white wine, lemon zest, salt, and pepper. Cook over low heat for 5 minutes. Stir in spinach, let wilt for 2 minutes and stir in shirataki fettuccine and salmon. Serve.

Nutrition: Calories 795; Net Carbs 9g; Fats 46g; Protein 72g

159) Easy Saucy Salmon with Tarragon

Preparation Time: approx. 20 minutes

Servings: 2

Ingredients:

✓ 2 salmon fillets
✓ 1 tbsp duck fat
✓ Salt and black pepper to taste

Directions:

❖ Season the salmon with salt and pepper. Melt the duck fat in a pan over medium heat. Add salmon and cook for 4 minutes on both sides; set aside. In the same pan, melt the butter and add the tarragon.

Ingredients:

✓ 2 tbsp butter
✓ ½ tsp tarragon, chopped
✓ ¼ cup heavy cream
❖ Cook for 30 seconds to infuse the flavors. Whisk in heavy cream and cook for 1 minute. Serve salmon topped with the sauce.

Nutrition: Calories 468; Net Carbs 1.5g; Fat 40g; Protein 22g

160) Best Cheesy Baked Trout with Zucchini

Preparation Time: approx. 40 minutes

Servings: 4

Ingredients:

✓ 4 deboned trout fillets
✓ 2 zucchinis, sliced
✓ 1 tbsp butter, melted

Directions:

❖ Preheat oven to 390 F. Brush the fish and zucchini slices with melted butter. Spread them in a greased baking dish. Mix the Greek yogurt with cheddar cheese in a bowl.

Ingredients:

✓ 1 cup Greek yogurt
✓ ¼ cup cheddar cheese, grated
✓ Grated Parmesan for topping
❖ Pour and smear the mixture on the fish and sprinkle with Parmesan cheese. Bake for 30 minutes until golden brown

Nutrition: Calories 362; Net Carbs 5.8g; Fat 23g; Protein 25g

161)   Best .Traditional Salmon Panzanella

Preparation   Time: approx.   25 minutes

Servings: 4

Ingredients:

- ✓ 1 lb skinned salmon, cut into 4 steaks each
- ✓ 8 black olives, pitted and chopped
- ✓ 1 cucumber, cubed
- ✓ Salt and black pepper to taste
- ✓ 1 tbsp capers, rinsed

Ingredients:

- ✓ 2 large tomatoes, diced
- ✓ 3 tbsp white wine vinegar
- ✓ ¼ cup thinly sliced red onions
- ✓ 3 tbsp olive oil
- ✓ 2 slices zero carb bread, cubed

Directions:

- ❖ Preheat grill to high. In a bowl, mix cucumber, black olives, salt, pepper, capers, tomatoes, white wine vinegar, onions, olive oil, and bread cubes. Let sit so the flavors to incorporate.

- ❖ Season the salmon with salt and pepper and grill it on both sides for 8 minutes. Serve the salmon steaks warm on a bed of the salad.

Nutrition: Calories 338; Net Carbs 3.1g; Fat 21g; Protein 28g

162)   Special Teriyaki Salmon with Steamed Broccoli

Preparation Time:approx. 30 min + chilling time

Servings: 4

Ingredients:

- ✓ ¼ cup grated Pecorino Romano cheese + some more
- ✓ 4 salmon fillets
- ✓ ½ cup teriyaki sauce

Ingredients:

- ✓ 1 bunch of broccoli rabe
- ✓ Salt and black pepper to taste

Directions:

- ❖ Cover the salmon with the teriyaki sauce and refrigerate for 30 minutes. Steam the broccoli rabe for 4-5 minutes until tender. Season with salt and pepper and set aside.

- ❖ Preheat oven to 400 F. Remove the salmon from the fridge and place in a greased baking dish. Bake in the oven for 14-16 minutes. Serve with steamed broccoli rabe.

Nutrition: Calories 354; Net Carbs 4g; Fat 17g; Protein 28g

163)   Easy Baked Salmon with Pistachio Crust

Preparation   Time: approx.   35 minutes

Servings: 4

Ingredients:

- ✓ 4 salmon fillets
- ✓ ¼ cup mayonnaise
- ✓ ½ cup ground pistachios
- ✓ 1 chopped shallot
- ✓ 2 tsp lemon zest

Ingredients:

- ✓ 1 tbsp olive oil
- ✓ A pinch of pepper
- ✓ 1 cup heavy cream

Directions:

- ❖ Preheat oven to 375 F. Spread mayonnaise on the fillets. Coat with ground pistachios. Place in a lined baking dish and bake for 15 minutes. Heat the olive oil in a saucepan and sauté shallot for 3 minutes

- ❖ Stir in heavy cream and lemon zest. Bring to a boil and cook until thickened. Pour the sauce over the salmon and serve.

Nutrition: Calories 563; Net Carbs 6g; Fat 47g; Protein 34g

164)   Rich Party Smoked Salmon Balls

Preparation Time: approx 30 minutes

Servings: 6

Ingredients:
- ✓ 12 oz sliced smoked salmon, finely chopped
- ✓ 1 parsnip, cooked and mashed
- ✓ Salt and chili pepper to taste
- ✓ 4 tbsp olive oil

Ingredients:
- ✓ 2 eggs, beaten
- ✓ 2 tbsp pesto sauce
- ✓ 1 tbsp pork rinds, crushed

Directions:
- ❖ In a bowl, add the salmon, eggs, pesto sauce, pork rinds, salt, and chili pepper. Mix well and make 6 compact balls.

- ❖ Heat olive oil in a skillet over medium heat and fry the balls for 3 minutes on each side until golden brown. Remove to a wire rack to cool. Serve warm.

Nutrition: Calories 254; Net Carbs 4.3g; Fat 18g; Protein 17g

165)   Italian Salmon Caesar Salad with Poached Eggs

Preparation Time: approx. 15 minutes

Servings: 4

Ingredients:
- ✓ ½ cup chopped smoked salmon
- ✓ 2 tbsp heinz low carb caesar dressing
- ✓ 3 cups water

Ingredients:
- ✓ 8 eggs
- ✓ 2 cups torn romaine lettuce
- ✓ 4 pancetta slices
- ❖ Poach the remaining eggs. Put the pancetta in a skillet and fry for 6 minutes, turning once. Allow cooling and chop into small pieces. Toss the lettuce, smoked salmon, pancetta, and caesar dressing in a salad bowl. Top with the eggs.

Directions:
- ❖ Boil water in a pot over medium heat. Crack each egg into a small bowl and gently slide into the water. Poach for 2-3 minutes, remove, and transfer to a plate.

Nutrition: Calories 260; Net Carbs 5g; Fat 21g; Protein 8g

166)   Special Mahi Mahi with Dill Sour Cream Topping

Preparation Time: approx. 30 minutes

Servings: 4

Ingredients:
- ✓ ½ cup grated Pecorino Romano cheese
- ✓ 1 cup sour cream
- ✓ ½ tbsp minced dill

Ingredients:
- ✓ ½ lemon, zested and juiced
- ✓ 4 mahi mahi fillets

Directions:
- ❖ Preheat oven to 400 F. Line a baking sheet with parchment paper. In a bowl, mix sour cream, dill, and lemon zest; set aside. Drizzle the mahi mahi with lemon juice and arrange on the baking sheet.

- ❖ Spread sour cream mixture on top and sprinkle with Pecorino Romano cheese. Bake for 15 minutes. Broil the top for 2 minutes until nicely brown. Serve with buttery green beans.

Nutrition: Calories 288; Net Carbs 1.2g; Fat 23g; Protein 16g

167)   Paleo Mediterranean Tilapia

Preparation Time: approx. 30 minutes

Servings: 4

Ingredients:
- ✓ 4 tilapia fillets
- ✓ 2 garlic cloves, minced
- ✓ ½ tsp dry oregano
- ✓ 14 oz canned diced tomatoes

Ingredients:
- ✓ 2 tbsp olive oil
- ✓ ½ red onion, chopped
- ✓ 1 tbsp fresh parsley, chopped
- ✓ ¼ cup kalamata olives
- ❖ Add olives and tilapia. Cook for 8 minutes. Serve topped with parsley.

Directions:
- ❖ Heat oil in a skillet over medium heat and cook onion for 3 minutes. Add garlic and oregano and cook for 30 seconds.
- ❖ Stir in tomatoes and bring the mixture to a boil. Reduce the heat and simmer for 5 minutes.

Nutrition: Calories 182; Net Carbs 6g; Fat 15g; Protein 23g

168)   Easy Paleo Lamb and Coconut Stew

Preparation Time: 1 hour 15 minutes

Servings: 4

Ingredients:
- ✓ 1 and ½ lb. lamb meat, diced
- ✓ 1 tbsp. coconut oil
- ✓ ½ red chili, seedless and chopped
- ✓ 1 brown onion, chopped
- ✓ 3 garlic cloves, minced
- ✓ 2 celery sticks, chopped
- ✓ 2 and ½ tsp. garam masala powder
- ✓ 1 tsp. fennel seeds
- ✓ Salt and black pepper to taste

Ingredients:
- ✓ 1 and ¼ tsp. turmeric
- ✓ 1 and ½ tsp. ghee
- ✓ 14 oz. canned coconut milk
- ✓ 1 and ½ tbsp. coconut milk
- ✓ 1 cup water
- ✓ 1 tbsp. lemon juice
- ✓ 2 carrots, chopped
- ✓ A handful parsley leaves, finely chopped

Directions:
- ❖ Heat up a pan with the oil over medium-high heat, add lamb, stir and brown for 4 minutes.
- ❖ Add celery, chili and onion, stir and cook 1 minute.
- ❖ Reduce heat to medium, add garam masala, garlic, ghee, fennel, and turmeric, stir and cook 1 minute.

- ❖ Add salt, pepper to the taste, tomato paste, coconut milk, and water, stir, bring to a boil, reduce heat to low, cover and cook for 1 hour.
- ❖ Add carrots and cook fro 40 minutes more, stirring from time to time.
- ❖ Add lemon juice and parsley, stir, take off heat, transfer to bowls and serve.
- ❖ Enjoy!

Nutrition: Calories 450 | Fat: 31g | Carbs: 40g |Protein: 50g | Fiber: 1g | Sugar: 0g

169) Special Paleo Veggie Stew

Preparation Time: 30 minutes

Servings: 4

Ingredients:
- ✓ 4 lb. mixed root vegetables (parsnips, carrots, rutabagas, potatoes, beets, celery root, turnips), chopped
- ✓ 6 tbsp. extra virgin olive oil
- ✓ 1 garlic head, cloves separated and peeled
- ✓ ½ cup yellow onion, chopped
- ✓ Salt and black pepper to taste

Directions:
- ❖ In a baking dish, mix all root vegetables with salt, pepper, half of the oil and garlic, toss to coat, introduce in the oven at 450 degrees G and roast them for 45 minutes.
- ❖ Heat up a pot with the rest of the oil over medium-high heat, add onions and cook for 2-3 minutes stirring often.
- ❖ Add tomato paste, stir and cook one more minute.

Ingredients:
- ✓ 28 oz. canned tomatoes, peeled and chopped
- ✓ 1 tbsp. tomato paste
- ✓ 2 cups kale leaves, torn
- ✓ 1 tsp. oregano, dried
- ✓ Tabasco sauce for serving

- ❖ Add tomatoes and their liquid, some salt and pepper and the oregano, stir, bring to a simmer, reduce heat to low and cook until veggies become roasted.
- ❖ Take root vegetables out of the oven, add them to the pot and stir.
- ❖ Add kale, stir and cook for 5 minutes.
- ❖ Add Tabasco sauce to the taste, mix, transfer to bowls and serve.
- ❖ Enjoy!

Nutrition: Calories 150 | Fat: 7g | Carbs: 17.2g | Protein: 2.4g | Fiber: 3.7g | Sugar: 0g

170) Easy Paleo French Chicken Stew

Preparation Time: 30 minutes

Servings: 4

Ingredients:
- ✓ 10 garlic cloves, peeled
- ✓ 30 black olives, pitted
- ✓ 2 lb. chicken pieces
- ✓ 2 cups chicken stock
- ✓ 28 oz. canned tomatoes, chopped

Directions:
- ❖ Heat up a pot with some olive oil over medium-high heat, add chicken pieces, salt, and pepper to the taste and cook for 4 minutes, stirring often.
- ❖ Add garlic, stir and brown for 2 minutes.
- ❖ Add chicken stock, tomatoes, olives, thyme, and rosemary, stir, cover pot and bake in the oven at 325 degrees for 1 hour.

Ingredients:
- ✓ 2 tbsp. rosemary, chopped
- ✓ 2 tbsp. parsley leaves, chopped
- ✓ 2 tbsp. basil leaves, chopped
- ✓ Salt and black pepper to taste
- ✓ A drizzle of extra virgin olive oil
- ❖ Add parsley and basil, mix, introduce in the oven again and bake for 45 more minutes.
- ❖ Leave stew to cool down for a few minutes, transfer to plates and serve.
- ❖ Enjoy!

Nutrition: Calories 300 | Fat: 48g | Carbs: 16g | Protein: 61g | Fiber: 6g | Sugar: 0g

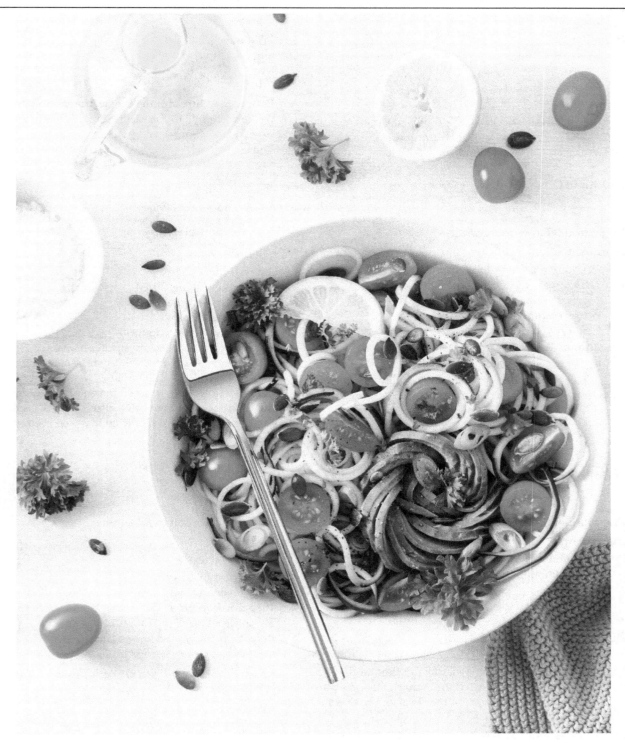

171) Mint ice cream

Preparation Time: 10 minutes + cooling time

Servings: 4

Ingredients:
- ✓ 2 avocados, pitted
- ✓ 1 ¼ cup coconut cream
- ✓ ½ tsp vanilla extract

Directions:
- ❖ In a blender, pour the avocado pulp, coconut cream, vanilla extract, erythritol and mint leaves. Process until the mixture is smooth.

Ingredients:
- ✓ 2 tbsp erythritol
- ✓ 2 tbsp chopped mint leaves

- ❖ Pour the mixture into the ice cream maker and freeze according to the manufacturer's instructions. When ready, remove and pour ice cream into a bowl.

Nutrition: Calories 370; Net carbohydrates 4g; Fat 38g; Protein 4g

172) Pizza with sweet onion and goat cheese

Preparation Time: 35 minutes

Servings: 4

Ingredients:
- ✓ 2 cups grated mozzarella cheese
- ✓ 2 tbsp cream cheese, softened
- ✓ 2 large eggs, beaten
- ✓ ⅓ cup almond flour
- ✓ 1 tsp dry Italian seasoning

Directions:
- ❖ Preheat oven to 390 F. Line a round pizza pan with baking paper. Microwave the mozzarella and cream cheeses for 1 minute. Remove and mix in the eggs, almond flour and Italian seasoning. Spread the mixture on the baking sheet and bake for 6 minutes.

Ingredients:
- ✓ 2 tbsp butter
- ✓ 2 red onions, thinly sliced
- ✓ 1 cup crumbled goat cheese
- ✓ 1 tbsp almond milk
- ✓ 1 cup curly endive, chopped
- ❖ Melt butter in a skillet and stir in onions, salt and pepper and cook over low heat and stirring often until caramelized, 15-20 minutes. In a bowl, mix the goat cheese with the almond milk and spread over the crust. Top with the caramelized onions. Bake for 10 minutes. Scatter curly endive over the top, slice and serve.

Nutrition: Calories 317; Net Carbs 3g; Fat 20g; Protein 28g

173) Pizza with spinach and olives

Preparation Time: 40 minutes

Servings: 4

Ingredients:
- ✓ 1 cup grated mozzarella cheese
- ✓ ½ cup almond flour
- ✓ ¼ tsp salt
- ✓ 2 tbsp ground psyllium husk
- ✓ 1 tbsp olive oil

Directions:
- ❖ Preheat oven to 390 F. Line a baking sheet with parchment paper. In a bowl, mix the almond flour, salt, psyllium husk, olive oil and water until a dough forms. Spread the dough on the sheet and bake for 10 minutes

Ingredients:
- ✓ 1 cup warm water
- ✓ ½ cup of tomato sauce
- ✓ ½ cup baby spinach
- ✓ 1 tsp dried oregano
- ✓ 3 tbsp sliced black olives
- ❖ Remove the crust and spread the tomato sauce on top. Add the spinach, mozzarella, oregano and olives. Bake for 15 minutes. Remove from oven, slice and serve warm.

Nutrition: Calories 195; Net Carbs 1.8g; Fat 8g; Protein 11g

174)   Tofu Nuggets with cilantro sauce

Preparation Time: 25 minutes   **Servings: 4**

Ingredients:

- ✓ 1 lime, ½ squeezed and ½ cut into wedges
- ✓ 1 ½ cups olive oil
- ✓ 28 ounces tofu, pressed and diced
- ✓ 1 egg, lightly beaten
- ✓ 1 cup golden flax seed meal

Directions:

- ❖ Heat the olive oil in a deep skillet. Coat the tofu cubes in the egg and then in the flaxseed meal. Fry until golden brown.

Ingredients:

- ✓ 1 ripe avocado, chopped
- ✓ ½ tbsp chopped cilantro
- ✓ Salt and black pepper to taste
- ✓ ½ tbsp olive oil

- ❖ Transfer to a plate. Place the avocado, cilantro, salt, pepper and lime juice in a blender; blend until smooth. Pour into a bowl, add the tofu nuggets and lime wedges to serve.

Nutrition: Calories 665; Net carbs 6.2g, fat 54g, protein 32g

175)   Spicy Brussels sprouts with carrots

Preparation Time: 15 minutes   **Servings: 4**

Ingredients:

- ✓ 1 pound Brussels sprouts
- ✓ ¼ cup olive oil
- ✓ 4 green onions, chopped

Directions:

- ❖ Sauté green onions in hot olive oil for 2 minutes. Sprinkle with salt and pepper and transfer to a plate. Cut the Brussels sprouts and split them in half.

Ingredients:

- ✓ 2 carrots, grated
- ✓ Salt and black pepper to taste
- ✓ Hot chili sauce
- ❖ Leave the small ones as whole. Pour the Brussels sprouts and carrots into the same saucepan and sauté until softened but al dente. Season to taste and toss with the onions. Cook for 3 minutes. Add chili sauce and serve.

Nutrition: Calories 198; Net carbohydrates 6.5g; Fat 14g; Protein 4.9g

176)   Zucchini-Cranberry Cake Squares

Preparation Time: 45 minutes   **Servings: 6**

Ingredients:

- ✓ 1 ¼ cups chopped zucchini
- ✓ 2 tbsp olive oil
- ✓ ½ cup dried cranberries
- ✓ 1 lemon, peeled
- ✓ 3 eggs

Directions:

- ❖ Preheat oven to 350 F. Line a square cake pan with baking paper. Combine the zucchini, olive oil, cranberries, lemon zest and eggs in a bowl until evenly combined.

Ingredients:

- ✓ 1 ½ cups almond flour
- ✓ ½ tsp baking powder
- ✓ 1 tsp cinnamon powder
- ✓ A pinch of salt

- ❖ Add the almond flour, baking powder, cinnamon powder and salt into the mixture. Pour the mixture into the cake pan and bake for 30 minutes. Remove from the oven, let cool in the cake pan for 10 minutes and transfer the cake to a wire rack to cool completely. Cut into squares and serve.

Nutrition: Calories 121; Net Carbs 2.5g, Fat 10g, Protein 4g

177) Fried rice egg with grilled cheese

Preparation Time: 10 minutes   **Servings: 4**

Ingredients:

- ✓ 2 cups cauliflower rice, steamed
- ✓ ½ pound halloumi, cut into ¼- to ½-inch slabs
- ✓ 1 tbsp ghee
- ✓ 4 eggs, beaten

Directions:

- ❖ Melt the ghee in a skillet and pour in the eggs. Rotate the pan to scatter the eggs and cook for 1 minute. Move the scrambled eggs to the side of the skillet, add the bell bell pepper and green beans and saute for 3 minutes. Pour in the cauli rice and cook for 2 minutes.

Ingredients:

- ✓ 1 green bell pepper, chopped
- ✓ ¼ cup green beans, chopped
- ✓ 1 tsp soy sauce
- ✓ 2 tbsp chopped parsley
- ❖ Add the soy sauce; combine evenly and cook for 2 minutes. Distribute to plates, garnish with parsley and set aside. Preheat a grill pan and grill halloumi cheese on both sides until cheese turns slightly brown. Place on the side of the rice and serve hot.

Nutrition: Calories 275; Net carbs 4.5g, fat 19g, protein 15g

178) Fake Mushroom Risotto

Preparation Time: 15 minutes   **Servings: 4**

Ingredients:

- ✓ 2 shallots, diced
- ✓ 3 tbsp olive oil
- ✓ ¼ cup vegetable stock
- ✓ ⅓ cup Parmesan cheese

Directions:

- ❖ Heat 2 tbsp oil in a saucepan, add mushrooms and cook over medium heat for 3 minutes.

Ingredients:

- ✓ 4 tbsp butter
- ✓ 3 tbsp chopped chives
- ✓ 2 pounds mushrooms, sliced
- ✓ 4 1/2 cups rinsed cauliflower
- ❖ Remove and set aside. Heat the remaining oil and cook the shallots for 2 minutes. Add the cauliflower and broth and cook until the liquid is absorbed. Stir in the rest of the ingredients.

Nutrition: Calories 264; Net carbs 8.4g; Fat 18g; Protein 11g

179) Eggplant pizza with cheese

Preparation Time: 40 minutes   **Servings: 2**

Ingredients:

- ✓ 6 ounces grated mozzarella cheese
- ✓ 2 tbsp cream cheese
- ✓ 2 tbsp Parmesan cheese
- ✓ 1 tsp oregano
- ✓ ½ cup almond flour
- ✓ 2 tbsp psyllium husk

Directions:

- ❖ Preheat oven to 400 F. Melt the mozzarella cheese in the microwave. Combine cream cheese, Parmesan cheese, oregano, almond flour and psyllium husk in a bowl. Add the melted mozzarella cheese and stir to combine.

Ingredients:

- ✓ 4 ounces grated cheddar cheese
- ✓ ¼ cup marinara sauce
- ✓ Eggplant, sliced
- ✓ 1 tomato, sliced
- ✓ 2 tbsp chopped basil
- ✓ 6 black olives
- ❖ Divide the dough into 2. Roll out the crusts into circles and place on a lined baking sheet. Bake for 10 minutes. Add the cheddar cheese, marinara, eggplant, tomato and basil. Return to oven and bake for 10 minutes. Serve with olives.

Nutrition: Calories 510; Net Carbs 3.7g; Fat 39g; Protein 31g

180)   Eggplant and Goat Cheese Pizza

Preparation Time: 45 minutes

Servings: 4

Ingredients:

- ✓ 4 tbsp olive oil
- ✓ 2 eggplants, sliced lengthwise
- ✓ 1 cup tomato sauce
- ✓ 2 garlic cloves, minced
- ✓ 1 red onion, sliced
- ✓ 12 ounces goat cheese, crumbled

Ingredients:

- ✓ Salt and black pepper to taste
- ✓ ½ tsp cinnamon powder
- ✓ 1 cup mozzarella cheese, shredded
- ✓ 2 tbsp oregano, chopped

Directions:

- ❖ Line a baking sheet with baking paper. Arrange eggplant slices on baking sheet and drizzle with a little olive oil. Bake for 20 minutes at 390 F. Heat the remaining olive oil in a skillet and sauté the garlic and onion for 3 minutes.

- ❖ Add goat cheese and tomato sauce and season with salt and pepper. Simmer for 10 minutes. Remove eggplant from oven and spread cheese sauce on top. Sprinkle with mozzarella cheese and oregano. Bake for 10 minutes more until cheese melts. Cut into slices and serve.

Nutrition: Calories 557; Net Carbs 8.3g; Fat 44g; Protein 33g

181)   Mushroom and broccoli pizza

Preparation Time: 25 minutes

Servings: 4

Ingredients:

- ✓ ½ cup almond flour
- ✓ ¼ tsp salt
- ✓ 2 tbsp ground psyllium husk
- ✓ 2 tbsp olive oil
- ✓ 1 cup fresh sliced mushrooms
- ✓ 1 white onion, thinly sliced

Ingredients:

- ✓ 3 cups broccoli florets
- ✓ 2 cloves garlic, minced
- ✓ ½ cup unsweetened pizza sauce
- ✓ 4 tomatoes, sliced
- ✓ 1 ½ cups mozzarella cheese, grated
- ✓ ⅓ cup grated Parmesan cheese
- ❖ Heat the remaining olive oil in a skillet and sauté mushrooms, onion, garlic and broccoli for 5 minutes. Spread the pizza sauce over the crust and top with the broccoli mixture, tomato, mozzarella and Parmesan. Bake for 5 minutes. Serve in slices.

Directions:

- ❖ Preheat oven to 390 F. Line a baking sheet with parchment paper. In a bowl, mix almond flour, salt, psyllium powder, 1 tbsp olive oil and 1 cup warm water until a dough forms. Spread the dough onto the pizza pan and bake for 10 minutes.

Nutrition: Calories 180; Net carbs 3.6g; Fat 9g; Protein 17g

182)   Tofu radish bowls

Preparation Time: 35 minutes

Servings: 4

Ingredients:

- ✓ ¼ cup baby mushrooms, chopped
- ✓ 2 yellow peppers, chopped
- ✓ 1 block of tofu (14 oz), cubed
- ✓ 1 tbsp + 1 tbsp olive oil
- ✓ 1 ½ cups shredded radishes

Ingredients:

- ✓ ½ cup chopped white onions
- ✓ 4 eggs
- ✓ 1/3 cup tomato sauce
- ✓ A handful of chopped parsley
- ✓ 1 avocado, and chopped
- ❖ Transfer to the top of a bowl of tofu hash and make the remaining eggs. Top the bowls with the tomato sauce, parsley and avocado. Serve.

Directions:

- ❖ Heat 1 tbsp olive oil in a skillet and add tofu, radishes, onions, mushrooms and peppers; cook for 10 minutes. Divide among 4 bowls. Heat the remaining oil in the skillet, crack an egg into the pan and cook until the white sets but the yolk is quite runny.

Nutrition: Calories 353; Net Carbs 5.9g, Fat 25g, Protein 19g

183) **Tomato & Mozzarella Caprese Bake**

Preparation Time: 25 minutes

Servings: 4

Ingredients:
- ✓ 4 tbsp olive oil
- ✓ 4 tomatoes, sliced
- ✓ 1 cup fresh mozzarella, sliced

Directions:
- ❖ In a baking dish, arrange the tomatoes and mozzarella slices. In a bowl, mix the pesto, mayonnaise and half of the Parmesan cheese; stir to combine.

Ingredients:
- ✓ 2 tbsp basil pesto
- ✓ 1 cup mayonnaise
- ✓ 2 ounces Parmesan cheese, grated
- ❖ Spread this mixture over the tomatoes and mozzarella and top with the remaining Parmesan cheese. Bake for 20 minutes at 360 F. Remove, let cool slightly and slice to serve.

Nutrition: Calories 420; Net Carbs 4.9g; Fat 36g; Protein 17g

184) **Cookies with heart of pistachio**

Preparation Time: 30 min + cooling time

Servings: 4

Ingredients:
- ✓ 1 cup butter, softened
- ✓ 2/3 cup sugar swerve
- ✓ 1 large egg, beaten
- ✓ 2 tsp pistachio extract

Directions:
- ❖ Add the butter and swerve sugar to a bowl and beat until smooth and creamy. Beat in the egg until combined. Stir in the pistachio extract and almond flour until a smooth dough forms. Wrap the dough in plastic wrap and chill for 10 minutes. Preheat oven to 350 F. Lightly dust a cutting board with almond flour. Unroll the dough and roll it out to a thickness of 2 inches.

Ingredients:
- ✓ 2 cups almond flour
- ✓ ½ cup dark chocolate
- ✓ 2 tbsp chopped pistachios

- ❖ Cut out as many cookies as you can get, while rolling back the scraps to make more cookies. Place the cookies on the baking sheet lined with parchment paper and bake for 15 minutes. Transfer to a wire rack to cool completely. Melt the dark chocolate in the microwave. Dip one side of each cookie into the melted chocolate. Garnish chocolate side with pistachios and let cool on a wire rack. Serve.

Nutrition: Calories 470; Net carbs 3.4g, fat 45g, protein 6.2g

185)   Avocado and tomato burritos

Preparation Time: 10 minutes

Servings: 4

Ingredients:
- ✓ 2 cups cauli rice
- ✓ 6 low carb tortillas
- ✓ 2 cups sour cream sauce

Ingredients:
- ✓ 1 ½ cups herbed tomato sauce
- ✓ 2 avocados, peeled, pitted and sliced

Directions:
- ❖ Pour cauli rice into a bowl, sprinkle with a little water, and microwave for 2 minutes to soften. On the tortillas, spread the sour cream and spread the salsa on top.

- ❖ Top with the cauli rice and spread the avocado evenly on top. Fold and tuck the burritos and cut in half. Serve.

Nutrition: Calories 303, Fat 25g, Net Carbs 6g, Protein 8g

186)   Creamy cucumber and avocado soup

Preparation Time: 15 minutes

Servings: 4

Ingredients:
- ✓ 4 large cucumbers, seeded and cut into pieces
- ✓ 1 large avocado, peeled and cut in half
- ✓ Salt and black pepper to taste
- ✓ 1 tbsp fresh cilantro, chopped
- ✓ 3 tbsp olive oil

Ingredients:
- ✓ 2 limes, squeezed
- ✓ 2 tbsp minced garlic
- ✓ 2 tomatoes, chopped
- ✓ 1 avocado, chopped for garnish

Directions:
- ❖ Pour cucumbers, avocado halves, salt, black pepper, olive oil, lime juice, cilantro, 2 cups water and garlic into food processor. Puree the ingredients for 2 minutes or until smooth.

- ❖ Pour mixture into a bowl and top with avocado and chopped tomatoes. Serve cold with zero carb bread.

Nutrition: Calories 170, Fat 7.4g, Net Carbs 4.1g, Protein 3.7g

187)   Cauliflower "couscous" with lemon and Halloumi

Preparation Time: 5 minutes

Servings: 4

Ingredients:
- ✓ 4 ounces of halloumi, sliced
- ✓ 2 tbsp olive oil
- ✓ 1 head of cauliflower, cut into florets
- ✓ ¼ cup chopped cilantro

Ingredients:
- ✓ ¼ cup chopped parsley
- ✓ ¼ cup chopped mint
- ✓ ½ lemon, squeezed
- ✓ Salt and black pepper to taste
- ✓ 1 avocado, sliced for garnish

Directions:
- ❖ Heat the olive oil in a skillet over medium heat. Add halloumi and fry for 2 minutes on each side until golden brown; set aside. Pour the cauli florets into a food processor and pulse until it crumbles and resembles couscous. Transfer to a bowl and steam in the microwave for 2 minutes.

- ❖ Remove the bowl from the microwave and allow the cauli to cool. Add the cilantro, parsley, mint, lemon juice, salt and pepper. Top the couscous with avocado slices and serve with grilled halloumi and vegetable sauce.

Nutrition: Calories 185, Fat 15.6g, Net Carbs 2.1g, Protein 12g

188) Zucchini lasagna with ricotta cheese and spinach

Preparation Time: 50 minutes

Servings: 4

Ingredients:

- ✓ 2 zucchini, sliced
- ✓ Salt and black pepper to taste
- ✓ 2 cups ricotta cheese

Directions:

- ❖ Preheat oven to 370°F. Place zucchini slices in a colander and sprinkle with salt. Let stand and drain liquid for 5 minutes and pat dry with paper towels. Mix the ricotta, mozzarella, salt and black pepper to combine evenly and spread ¼ cup of the mixture over the bottom of the baking dish.
- ❖ Arrange ⅓ of the zucchini slices on top, spread 1 cup of the tomato sauce, and scatter ⅓ cup of the spinach on top.

Ingredients:

- ✓ 2 cups shredded mozzarella cheese
- ✓ 3 cups tomato sauce
- ✓ 1 cup spinach
- ❖ Repeat the layering process two more times to run out of ingredients, finally making sure to layer with the last ¼ cup of cheese mixture.
- ❖ Grease one end of the aluminum foil with cooking spray and cover the baking sheet with the foil. Bake for 35 minutes, remove the foil and bake further for 5-10 minutes or until the cheese has a nice golden brown color. Remove dish, let rest for 5 minutes, make lasagna slices and serve warm.

189) Briam with tomato sauce

Preparation Time: 40 minutes

Servings: 4

Ingredients:

- ✓ 3 tbsp olive oil
- ✓ 1 large eggplant, halved and sliced
- ✓ 1 large onion, thinly sliced
- ✓ 3 garlic cloves, sliced
- ✓ 2 tomatoes, diced
- ✓ 1 rutabaga, diced

Directions:

- ❖ Preheat oven to 400°F. Heat the olive oil in a skillet over medium heat and fry the eggplant and zucchini slices for 6 minutes until golden brown. Remove them to a casserole dish and arrange them in a single layer.

Ingredients:

- ✓ 1 cup unsweetened tomato sauce
- ✓ 4 zucchini, sliced
- ✓ ¼ cup water
- ✓ Salt and black pepper to taste
- ✓ ¼ tsp dried oregano
- ✓ 2 tbsp fresh parsley, chopped
- ❖ Sauté the onion and garlic in the oil for 3 minutes. Remove to a bowl. Add the tomatoes, rutabaga, tomato sauce and water and mix well. Stir in salt, pepper, oregano and parsley. Pour the mixture over the eggplant and zucchini. Place the dish in the oven and bake for 25-30 minutes. Serve the briam hot.

Nutrition: Calories Calories 365, Fat 12g, Net Carbohydrates 12.5g, Protein 11.3g

190) Creamy vegetable stew

Preparation Time: 25 minutes

Servings: 4

Ingredients:

- ✓ 2 tbsp ghee
- ✓ 1 tbsp onion and garlic puree
- ✓ 2 medium carrots, shredded
- ✓ 1 head of cauliflower, cut into florets

Directions:

- ❖ Melt ghee in a saucepan over medium heat and sauté onion and garlic puree to be fragrant, 2 minutes. Stir

Ingredients:

- ✓ 2 cups green beans, cut in half
- ✓ Salt and black pepper to taste
- ✓ 1 cup water
- ✓ 1 ½ cups heavy cream
- ❖ Pour in water, stir again and cook over low heat for 15 minutes. Stir in the heavy cream to incorporate and turn off the heat. Serve the stew with almond flour bread.

in carrots, cauliflower and green beans for 5 minutes. Season with salt and black pepper.

Nutrition: Calories 310, fat 26.4g, net carbs 6g, protein 8g

191) Tempeh kabobs with vegetables

Preparation Time: 30 minutes + cooling time

Servings: 4

Ingredients:
- ✓ 2 tbsp ghee
- ✓ 1 tbsp onion and garlic puree
- ✓ 2 medium carrots, shredded
- ✓ 1 head of cauliflower, cut into florets

Ingredients:
- ✓ 2 cups green beans, cut in half
- ✓ Salt and black pepper to taste
- ✓ 1 cup water
- ✓ 1 ½ cups heavy cream
- ❖ Pour in water, stir again and cook over low heat for 15 minutes. Stir in the heavy cream to incorporate and turn off the heat. Serve the stew with almond flour bread.

Directions:
- ❖ Melt ghee in a saucepan over medium heat and sauté onion and garlic puree to be fragrant, 2 minutes. Stir in carrots, cauliflower and green beans for 5 minutes. Season with salt and black pepper.

Nutrition: Calories Calories 228, Fat 15g, Net Carbohydrates 3.6g, Protein 13.2g

192) Tempeh kabobs with vegetables

Preparation Time: 30 minutes + cooling time

Servings: 4

Ingredients:
- ✓ 1 yellow bell pepper, cut into pieces
- ✓ 10 ounces tempeh, cut into pieces
- ✓ 1 red onion, cut into pieces

Ingredients:
- ✓ 1 red bell bell pepper, cut into pieces
- ✓ 2 tbsp olive oil
- ✓ 1 cup unsweetened barbecue sauce
- ❖ Preheat grill to 350°F. Thread the tempeh, yellow bell pepper, red bell pepper and onion onto skewers. Brush the grill grate with olive oil, place the skewers on and brush with the barbecue sauce. Cook skewers for 3 minutes on each side, rotating and brushing with more barbecue sauce. Serve.

Directions:
- ❖ Bring the 1 ½ cups of water to a boil in a pot over medium heat, and once it's cooked, turn off the heat and add the tempeh. Cover the pot and allow the tempeh to steam for 5 minutes to remove the bitterness. Drain. Pour barbecue sauce into a bowl, add tempeh and coat with sauce. Refrigerate for 2 hours.

Nutrition: Calories Calories 228, Fat 15g, Net Carbohydrates 3.6g, Protein 13.2g

193) Cauliflower and Gouda Cheese Casserole

Preparation Time: 25 minutes

Servings: 4

Ingredients:
- ✓ 2 heads of cauliflower, cut into florets
- ✓ 2 tbsp olive oil
- ✓ 2 tbsp melted butter
- ✓ 1 white onion, chopped

Ingredients:
- ✓ Salt and black pepper to taste
- ✓ ¼ cup almond milk
- ✓ ½ cup almond flour
- ✓ 1 ½ cups gouda cheese, grated
- ❖ Cook over low heat for 3 minutes. Mix the melted butter with the almond flour. Stir in the cauliflower and half of the cheese. Sprinkle the top with the remaining cheese and bake for 10 minutes until the cheese is melted and golden brown on top. Plate the oven and serve with the salad.

Directions:
- ❖ Preheat oven to 350°F. Place cauli florets in a large microwave-safe bowl. Sprinkle with a little water and steam in the microwave for 4 to 5 minutes. Heat the olive oil in a saucepan over medium heat and sauté

the onion for 3 minutes. Add the cauliflower, season with salt and pepper and stir in the almond milk.

Nutrition: Calories 215, Fat 15g, Net Carbs 4g, Protein 12g

194) Roasted Asparagus with Spicy Eggplant Sauce

Preparation Time: 35 minutes   **Servings: 6**

Ingredients:
- ✓ 1 ½ pounds asparagus, chopped
- ✓ ¼ cup + 2 tbsp olive oil
- ✓ ½ tsp paprika
- ✓ Eggplant Sauce
- ✓ 1 pound of eggplant
- ✓ ½ cup shallots, chopped

Ingredients:
- ✓ 2 cloves garlic, minced
- ✓ 1 tbsp fresh lemon juice
- ✓ ½ tsp chili pepper
- ✓ Salt and black pepper to taste
- ✓ ¼ cup fresh cilantro, chopped

Directions:
- ❖ Preheat oven to 390°F. Line a parchment paper on a baking sheet. Add the asparagus. Season with 2 tbsp olive oil, paprika, black pepper and salt. Roast until cooked through, 9 minutes. Remove.
- ❖ Place the eggplant on a cookie sheet lined baking sheet. Bake in the oven for about 20 minutes.

- ❖ Allow eggplant to cool. Peel them and discard the stems. Heat the remaining olive oil in a skillet over medium heat and add the garlic and shallots. Sauté for 3 minutes until tender.
- ❖ In a food processor, put together the black pepper, roasted eggplant, salt, lemon juice, shallot mixture, and red pepper. Add the cilantro and serve alongside the roasted asparagus spears.

Nutrition: Calories 149; Fat: 12.1g, Net Carbohydrates: 9g, Protein: 3.6g

195) Cook the squash

Preparation Time: 45 minutes   **Servings: 6**

Ingredients:
- ✓ 3 large pumpkins, peeled and sliced
- ✓ 1 cup almond flour
- ✓ 1 cup grated mozzarella cheese

Ingredients:
- ✓ 3 tbsp olive oil
- ✓ ½ cup fresh parsley, chopped

Directions:
- ❖ Preheat oven to 350°F. Arrange the squash slices in a baking dish and drizzle with olive oil.

- ❖ Bake for 35 minutes. Mix almond flour, mozzarella cheese and parsley and pour over squash. Return to oven and bake for another 5 minutes until top is golden brown. Serve warm.

Nutrition: Calories 125, Fat 4.8g, Net Carbs 5.7g, Protein 2.7g

196) Cremini Mushroom Stroganoff

Preparation Time: 25 minutes   **Servings: 4**

Ingredients:
- ✓ 3 tbsp butter
- ✓ 1 white onion, chopped
- ✓ 4 cups cremini mushrooms, diced

Ingredients:
- ✓ ½ cup heavy cream
- ✓ ½ cup Parmesan cheese, grated
- ✓ 1 ½ tbsp dried mixed herbs
- ❖ Cook for 10-15 minutes until the water reduces slightly. Pour in the heavy cream and Parmesan cheese. Stir to dissolve the cheese. Add the dried herbs and season. Simmer for 5 minutes. Serve hot.

Directions:
- ❖ Melt the butter in a saucepan over medium heat and sauté the onion for 3 minutes until soft. Add the mushrooms and cook until tender, about 5 minutes. Add 2 cups of water and bring to a boil.

Nutrition: Calories 284, Fat 28g, Net Carbs 1.5g, Protein 8g

197) Portobello Mushroom Burger

Preparation Time: 15 minutes

Servings: 4

Ingredients:

- ✓ 8 large portobello mushroom caps
- ✓ 1 minced garlic clove
- ✓ ½ cup of mayonnaise
- ✓ ½ tsp salt
- ✓ 4 tbsp olive oil
- ✓ ½ cup roasted red peppers, sliced

Directions:

- ❖ Preheat a grill over medium-high heat. In a bowl, crush the garlic with the salt using the back of a spoon. Stir in half the oil and brush the mushrooms and halloumi cheese with the mixture.
- ❖ Place the "sandwiches" on the skillet and grill them on both sides for 8 minutes until tender.

Ingredients:

- ✓ 2 medium tomatoes, chopped
- ✓ 4 halloumi slices, half-inch thick
- ✓ 1 tbsp red wine vinegar
- ✓ 2 tbsp Kalamata olives, chopped
- ✓ ½ tsp dried oregano
- ✓ 2 cups spinach
- ❖ Add the halloumi cheese slices to the grill. Cook for 2 minutes per side or until golden brown marks appear on the grill.
- ❖ In a bowl, mix red peppers, tomatoes, olives, vinegar, oregano, spinach and remaining olive oil; toss to coat. Spread mayonnaise on 4 mushroom "sandwiches", top with a slice of halloumi, a scoop of greens and top with remaining mushrooms. Serve and enjoy!

Nutrition: Calories 339, Fat 29.4g, Net Carbs 3.5g, Protein 10g

198) Sriracha tofu with yogurt sauce

Preparation Time: 40 minutes

Servings: 4

Ingredients:

- ✓ 12 ounces tofu, pressed and sliced
- ✓ 1 cup green onions, chopped
- ✓ 1 clove garlic, minced
- ✓ 2 tbsp vinegar
- ✓ 1 tbsp sriracha sauce
- ✓ 2 tbsp olive oil

Directions:

- ❖ Place the tofu slices, garlic, sriracha sauce, vinegar and green onions in a bowl. Let stand for 30 minutes. Place a nonstick skillet over medium heat and add oil to heat. Cook the tofu for 5 minutes until golden brown.

Ingredients:

- ✓ Yogurt Sauce
- ✓ 2 cloves garlic, crushed
- ✓ 2 tbsp fresh lemon juice
- ✓ Salt and black pepper to taste
- ✓ 1 tsp fresh dill
- ✓ 1 cup Greek yogurt
- ✓ 1 cucumber, shredded
- ❖ To make the sauce: In a bowl, mix garlic, salt, yogurt, black pepper, lemon juice and dill. Add shredded cucumber while stirring to combine. Serve tofu with a spoonful of yogurt sauce.

Nutrition: Calories 351; Fat: 25.9g, Net Carbohydrates: 8.1g, Protein: 17.5g

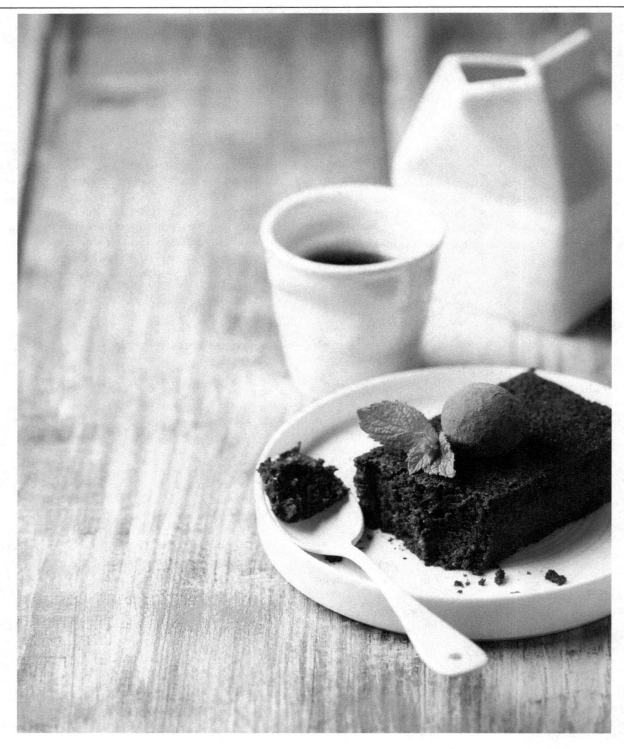

199)   Spinach and Turnip Salad with Bacon

Preparation Time: 40   minutes   **Servings: 4**

Ingredients:

- ✓   2 turnips, cut into wedges
- ✓   1 tsp olive oil
- ✓   1 cup baby spinach, chopped
- ✓   3 radishes, sliced
- ✓   3 slices turkey bacon
- ✓   4 tbsp sour cream

Directions:

- ❖   Preheat oven to 400°F. Line a baking sheet with parchment paper, toss the turnips with salt and black pepper, drizzle with olive oil and bake for 25 minutes, turning halfway through. Allow to cool.

Ingredients:

- ✓   2 tbsp mustard seed
- ✓   1 tsp Dijon mustard
- ✓   1 tbsp red wine vinegar
- ✓   Salt and black pepper to taste
- ✓   1 tbsp chopped chives

- ❖   Spread the spinach in the bottom of a salad bowl and top with the radishes. Remove the turnips to the salad bowl. Fry the bacon in a skillet over medium heat until crispy, about 5 minutes.
- ❖   Mix sour cream, mustard seeds, mustard, vinegar and salt with the bacon. Add a little water to deglaze the bottom of the pan. Pour the bacon mixture over the vegetables and scatter the chives. Serve.

Nutrition: Calories 193, Fat 18.3g, Net Carbohydrates 3.1g, Protein 9.5g

200)   Chicken Salad with Grapefruit and Cashews

Preparation Time: 30 minutes +
marinating time   **Servings: 4**

Ingredients:

- ✓   1 grapefruit, peeled and segmented
- ✓   1 chicken breast
- ✓   4 green onions, sliced
- ✓   10 ounces baby spinach
- ✓   2 tbsp cashews

Directions:

- ❖   Toast cashews in a dry skillet over high heat for 2 minutes, shaking often. Set aside to cool, then cut them into small pieces. Preheat the grill to medium heat. Season the chicken with salt and pepper and brush it with a little olive oil.

Ingredients:

- ✓   1 red chili pepper, thinly sliced
- ✓   1 lemon, squeezed
- ✓   3 tbsp olive oil
- ✓   Salt and black pepper to taste

- ❖   Grill for 4 minutes per side. Remove to a plate and let it rest for a few minutes before slicing.
- ❖   Arrange the spinach and green onions on a serving platter. Season with salt, remaining olive oil and lemon juice. Stir to coat. Top with the chicken, chili and chicken. Sprinkle with cashews and serve.

Nutrition: Calories 178, Fat: 13.5g, Net carbohydrates: 3.2g, Protein: 9.1g

201) Cobb Salad with Blue Cheese Dressing

Preparation Time: 30 minutes

Ingredients:

- ✓ Dressing
- ✓ ½ cup buttermilk
- ✓ 1 cup mayonnaise
- ✓ 2 tbsp Worcestershire sauce
- ✓ ½ cup sour cream
- ✓ 1 cup blue cheese, crumbled
- ✓ 2 tbsp chives, chopped
- ✓ Salad
- ✓ 6 eggs
- ✓ 2 chicken breasts

Directions:

- ❖ In a bowl, whisk buttermilk, mayonnaise, Worcestershire sauce and sour cream. Stir in the blue cheese and chives. Refrigerate to chill until ready to use. Bring eggs to boil in salted water over medium heat for 10 minutes. Transfer to an ice bath to cool. Peel and chop. Set aside.
- ❖ Preheat a grill pan over high heat. Season chicken with salt and pepper. Grill for 3 minutes on each side. Remove to a plate to cool for 3 minutes and cut into pieces.

Servings: 6

Ingredients:

- ✓ 5 strips of bacon
- ✓ 1 iceberg lettuce, chopped
- ✓ Salt and black pepper to taste
- ✓ 1 romaine lettuce, cut into pieces
- ✓ 1 bibb lettuce, core, leaves removed
- ✓ 2 avocados, pitted and diced
- ✓ 2 large tomatoes, chopped
- ✓ ½ cup blue cheese, crumbled
- ✓ 2 shallots, chopped

- ❖ . Fry the bacon in the same skillet until crispy, about 6 minutes. Remove, let cool for 2 minutes and cut into pieces.
- ❖ Arrange the lettuce leaves in a salad bowl and, in individual piles, add the avocado, tomatoes, eggs, bacon and chicken. Sprinkle the salad with the blue cheese, scallions and black pepper. Drizzle the blue cheese dressing over the salad and serve with low carb bread.

Nutrition: Calories 122, Fat 14g, Net Carbs 2g, Protein 23g

202) Green mackerel salad

Preparation Time: 25 minutes

Ingredients:

- ✓ 4 oz smoked mackerel, flaked
- ✓ 2 eggs
- ✓ 1 tbsp coconut oil
- ✓ 1 cup green beans, chopped
- ✓ 1 avocado, sliced

Directions:

- ❖ In a bowl, whisk together the lemon juice, olive oil, salt and pepper. Set aside. Cook green beans in boiling salted water over medium heat for about 3 minutes. Remove with a slotted spoon and let cool.

Servings: 4

Ingredients:

- ✓ 4 cups mixed salad
- ✓ 2 tbsp olive oil
- ✓ 1 tbsp lemon juice
- ✓ Salt and black pepper to taste

- ❖ Add the eggs to the pot and cook for 8-10 minutes. Transfer the eggs to an ice water bath, peel the shells and slice. Place the mixed green salad in a serving bowl and add the green beans and smoked mackerel. Pour in the dressing and toss to coat. Top with sliced egg and avocado and serve.

Nutrition: Calories 356, Fat: 31.9g, Net Carbs: 0.8g, Protein: 1.3g

203)   Grilled Steak Salad with Pickled Peppers

Preparation Time: 15 minutes   **Servings: 4**

Ingredients:

- ✓ ½ lb skirt steak, sliced
- ✓ Salt and black pepper to taste
- ✓ 3 tbsp olive oil
- ✓ 1 head romaine lettuce, torn

Directions:

- ❖ Brush the steak slices with olive oil and season them with salt and black pepper on both sides. Heat a grill pan over high heat and cook the steaks on each side for about 5-6 minutes. Remove to a bowl.

Nutrition: Calories 315, Fat 26g, Net Carbs 2g, Protein 18g

Ingredients:

- ✓ 3 pickled peppers, chopped
- ✓ 2 tbsp red wine vinegar
- ✓ ½ cup queso fresco, crumbled
- ✓ 1 tbsp green olives, pitted, sliced
- ❖ Mix the lettuce, pickled peppers, remaining olive oil and vinegar in a salad bowl. Add beef and sprinkle with queso fresco and green olives. Serve.

204)   Cauliflower salad with shrimp and avocado

Preparation Time: 30 minutes   **Servings: 6**

Ingredients:

- ✓ 1 head cauliflower, florets only
- ✓ 1 pound medium shrimp, shelled
- ✓ ¼ cup + 1 tbsp olive oil
- ✓ 1 avocado, chopped

Directions:

- ❖ Heat 1 tbsp olive oil in a skillet and cook the shrimp for 8 minutes. Microwave the cauliflower for 5 minutes

Ingredients:

- ✓ 2 tbsp fresh dill, chopped
- ✓ ¼ cup lemon juice
- ✓ 2 tbsp lemon zest
- ✓ Salt and black pepper to taste
- ❖ Place the shrimp, cauliflower, and avocado in a bowl. Whisk the remaining olive oil, lemon zest, juice, dill, salt and pepper in another bowl. Pour over the dressing, toss to combine and serve immediately.

Nutrition: Calories 214, Fat: 17g, Net Carbs: 5g, Protein: 15g

205)   Caesar Salad with Smoked Salmon and Poached Eggs

Preparation Time: 15 minutes   **Servings: 4**

Ingredients:

- ✓ 8 eggs
- ✓ 2 cups torn romaine lettuce
- ✓ ½ cup smoked salmon, chopped

Directions:

- ❖ Bring a pot of water to a boil and pour in the vinegar. Crack each egg into a small bowl and gently slide it into the water. Soak for 2 to 3 minutes, remove with a slotted spoon and transfer to a paper towel to remove excess water and plate. Poach the remaining 7 eggs.

Nutrition: Calories 260, Fat 21g, Net Carbs 5g, Protein 8g

Ingredients:

- ✓ 6 slices of bacon
- ✓ 2 tbsp low-carb Caesar dressing
- ✓ 1 tbsp white wine vinegar
- ❖ Place the bacon in a skillet and fry it over medium heat until browned and crispy, about 6 minutes, turning once. Remove, let cool and cut into small pieces. Mix the lettuce, smoked salmon, bacon and Caesar dressing in a salad bowl. Top with two eggs each and serve immediately or chilled.

206) Bacon and Spinach Salad

Preparation Time: 20 minutes

Servings: 4

Ingredients:

- ✓ 1 avocado, chopped
- ✓ 1 avocado, sliced
- ✓ 1 spring onion, sliced
- ✓ 4 slices bacon, chopped
- ✓ 2 cups spinach
- ✓ 2 small heads of lettuce, chopped

Directions:

- ❖ Place a skillet over medium heat and cook the bacon for 5 minutes until crispy. Remove to a paper towel-lined plate to drain. Boil the eggs in boiling salted water for 10 minutes. Let them cool, peel and chop them.

Ingredients:

- ✓ 2 eggs
- ✓ 3 tbsp olive oil
- ✓ 1 tbsp Dijon mustard
- ✓ 1 tbsp apple cider vinegar
- ✓ Salt to taste

- ❖ Combine the spinach, lettuce, eggs, chopped avocado and spring onion in a large bowl. Whisk together the olive oil, mustard, apple cider vinegar and salt in another bowl. Pour the dressing over the salad and toss to combine. Top with the sliced avocado and bacon and serve.

Nutrition: Calories 350, Fat: 33g, Net Carbs: 3.4g, Protein: 7g

207) Brussels Sprouts Salad with Pecorino Cheese

Preparation Time: 35 minutes

Servings: 6

Ingredients:

- ✓ 2 lb Brussels sprouts, halved
- ✓ 3 tbsp olive oil
- ✓ Salt and black pepper to taste

Directions:

- ❖ Preheat the oven to 400°F. Toss brussels sprouts with olive oil, salt, black pepper and balsamic vinegar in a bowl. Spread on a baking sheet in an even layer.

Ingredients:

- ✓ 2 tbsp balsamic vinegar
- ✓ ¼ head red cabbage, shredded
- ✓ 1 cup Pecorino cheese, shredded
- ❖ Bake until tender on the inside and crisp on the outside, about 20-25 minutes. Transfer to a salad bowl and add the red cabbage. Stir until well combined. Sprinkle with cheese, divide salad on serving plates and serve.

Nutrition: Calories 210, Fat 18g, Net Carbs 6g, Protein 4g

208) Pork Burger Salad with Yellow Cheddar

Preparation Time: 25 minutes

Servings: 4

Ingredients:

- ✓ ½ pound ground pork
- ✓ Salt and black pepper to taste
- ✓ 2 tbsp olive oil
- ✓ 2 hearts of romaine lettuce, torn

Directions:

- ❖ Season the pork with salt and black pepper, mix it, and make medium-sized patties. Heat the butter in a skillet over medium heat and fry the patties on both sides for 10 minutes until golden brown and cooked through on the inside.

Ingredients:

- ✓ 2 firm tomatoes, sliced
- ✓ ¼ red onion, sliced
- ✓ 3 ounces yellow cheddar cheese, grated
- ✓ 2 tbsp butter
- ❖ Transfer to a rack to drain off the oil. Once cooled, cut into quarters.
- ❖ Mix the lettuce, tomatoes, and red onion in a salad bowl, drizzle with olive oil and salt. Stir and add the pork on top. Top with cheese and serve.

Nutrition: Calories 310, Fat 23g, Net Carbs 2g, Protein 22g

209) Italian style green salad

Preparation Time: 15 minutes

Servings: 4

Ingredients:
- ✓ 2 (8 oz) package mixed salad
- ✓ 8 strips of bacon
- ✓ 1 cup gorgonzola cheese, crumbled

Directions:
- ❖ Fry the bacon strips in a skillet over medium heat for 6 minutes, until golden brown and crispy. Remove to a paper towel-lined plate to drain. Chop when cooled. Pour the green salad into a serving bowl.

Ingredients:
- ✓ 1 tbsp white wine vinegar
- ✓ 3 tbsp extra virgin olive oil
- ✓ Salt and black pepper to taste
- ❖ In a small bowl, whisk the white wine vinegar, olive oil, salt and pepper. Drizzle the dressing over the salad and toss to coat. Top with gorgonzola cheese and bacon. Divide salad among plates and serve.

Nutrition: Calories 205, Fat 20g, Net Carbs 2g, Protein 4g

210) Broccoli Salad Salad with Mustard Vinaigrette

Preparation Time: 10 minutes

Servings: 6

Ingredients:
- ✓ ½ tsp granulated sugar swerve
- ✓ 1 tbsp Dijon mustard
- ✓ 2 tbsp olive oil
- ✓ 4 cups broccoli salad
- ✓ ⅓ cup mayonnaise

Directions:
- ❖ In a bowl, place the mayonnaise, Dijon mustard, sugar swerve, olive oil, celery seeds, vinegar and salt and whisk until well combined.

Ingredients:
- ✓ 1 tsp celery seeds
- ✓ 2 tbsp slivered almonds
- ✓ 1 ½ tbsp apple cider vinegar
- ✓ Salt to taste

- ❖ Place the broccoli salad in a large salad bowl. Pour the vinaigrette over the top. Stir to coat. Sprinkle with slivered almonds and serve immediately.

Nutrition: Calories 110, Fat: 10g, Net Carbs: 2g, Protein: 3g

211) Warm Artichoke Salad

Preparation Time: 30 minutes

Servings: 4

Ingredients:
- ✓ 6 baby artichokes
- ✓ 6 cups water
- ✓ 1 tbsp lemon juice
- ✓ ¼ cup cherry peppers, halved
- ✓ ¼ cup pitted olives, sliced
- ✓ ¼ cup olive oil

Directions:
- ❖ Combine the water and salt in a saucepan over medium heat. Trim and halve the artichokes. Add them to the pot and bring to a boil. Lower the heat and simmer for 20 minutes until tender.

Ingredients:
- ✓ ¼ tsp lemon zest
- ✓ 2 tbsp balsamic vinegar, unsweetened
- ✓ 1 tbsp chopped dill
- ✓ Salt and black pepper to taste
- ✓ 1 tbsp capers
- ✓ ¼ tsp caper brine
- ❖ Combine the rest of the ingredients, except the olives, in a bowl. Drain and arrange the artichokes on a serving platter. Pour prepared mixture over them; toss to combine well. Serve topped with the olives.

Nutrition: Calories 170, Fat: 13g, Net carbs: 5g, Protein: 1g

212)   Squid salad with cucumbers and chili sauce

Preparation Time: 30 minutes

Servings: 4

Ingredients:
- ✓ 4 tubes of squid, cut into strips
- ✓ ½ cup mint leaves
- ✓ 2 cucumbers, halved, cut into strips
- ✓ ½ cup cilantro, stalks reserved
- ✓ ½ red onion, finely sliced
- ✓ Salt and black pepper to taste

Ingredients:
- ✓ 1 tsp fish sauce
- ✓ 1 red chili pepper, coarsely chopped
- ✓ 1 garlic clove
- ✓ 2 limes, squeezed
- ✓ 1 tbsp fresh parsley, chopped
- ✓ 1 tsp olive oil

Directions:
- ❖ In a salad bowl, mix mint leaves, cucumber strips, cilantro leaves and red onion. Season with salt, black pepper and a little olive oil; set aside. In a mortar, pound the cilantro stalks and red pepper to form a paste using the pestle. Add the fish sauce and lime juice and stir with the pestle.

- ❖ Heat a frying pan over medium heat. Brown the squid on both sides until lightly browned, about 5 minutes. Pour the calamari over the salad and drizzle with the chili dressing. Stir to coat, garnish with parsley and serve.

Nutrition: Calories 318, Fat 22.5g, Net Carbohydrates 2.1g, Protein 24.6g

213)   Mozzarella and tomato salad with anchovies and olives

Preparation Time: 10 minutes

Servings: 2

Ingredients:
- ✓ 1 large tomato, sliced
- ✓ 4 basil leaves
- ✓ 8 slices of mozzarella
- ✓ 2 tbsp olive oil

Directions:
- ❖ Arrange the tomato slices on a serving platter. Place the mozzarella slices on top and top with the basil.

Ingredients:
- ✓ 2 canned anchovies, chopped
- ✓ 1 tsp balsamic vinegar
- ✓ 4 black olives, pitted and sliced
- ✓ Salt to taste
- ❖ Add the anchovies and olives on top. Drizzle with olive oil and vinegar. Sprinkle with salt and serve.

Nutrition: Calories 430, Fat: 26.8g, Net Carbohydrates: 2.4g, Protein:38.8g

214)   Strawberry salad with cheese and almonds

Preparation Time: 20 minutes

Servings: 2

Ingredients:
- ✓ 4 cups cabbage, chopped
- ✓ 4 strawberries, sliced
- ✓ ½ cup almonds, slivered

Directions:
- ❖ Preheat oven to 400°F. Arrange grated goat cheese in two circles on two pieces of parchment paper. Place in the oven and bake for 10 minutes. Find two equal bowls, place them upside down and carefully place the parchment paper on top to give the cheese a bowl-like shape.

Ingredients:
- ✓ 1 ½ cups hard goat cheese, grated
- ✓ 4 tbsp raspberry vinaigrette
- ✓ Salt and black pepper to taste
- ❖ Let cool like this for 15 minutes.
- ❖ Divide the cabbage between the bowls, sprinkle with salt and pepper, and drizzle with the vinaigrette. Stir to coat. Top with almonds and strawberries. Serve immediately.

Nutrition: Calories 445, Fat: 34.2g, Net Carbohydrates: 5.3g, Protein: 33g

215)   Spring salad with cheese balls

Preparation Time: 20 minutes

Servings: 6

Ingredients:
- ✓ Cheese balls
- ✓ 3 eggs
- ✓ 1 cup feta cheese, crumbled
- ✓ ½ cup Pecorino cheese, crumbled
- ✓ 1 cup Almond Flour
- ✓ 1 tbsp flax meal
- ✓ Salt and black pepper to taste
- ✓ Salad
- ✓ 1 head Iceberg lettuce, leaves pulled apart
- ✓ ½ cup cucumber, thinly sliced

Ingredients:
- ✓ 2 tomatoes, seeded and chopped
- ✓ ½ cup red onion, thinly sliced
- ✓ ½ cup radishes, thinly sliced
- ✓ ⅓ cup mayonnaise
- ✓ 1 tsp mustard
- ✓ 1 tsp paprika
- ✓ 1 tsp oregano
- ✓ Salt to taste

Directions:
- ❖ Preheat oven to 390°F. In a bowl, mix all the ingredients for the cheese balls. Form balls with the mixture. Place the balls on a lined baking sheet. Bake for 10 minutes until crispy.

- ❖ Arrange lettuce leaves on a large salad plate. Add radishes, tomatoes, cucumbers and red onion. In a small bowl, mix mayonnaise, paprika, salt, oregano and mustard. Sprinkle the mixture over the vegetables. Add cheese balls on top and serve.

Nutrition: Calories: 234; Fat 16.7g, Net Carbohydrates 7.9g, Protein 12.4g

216)   Mediterranean Salad

Preparation Time: 10 minutes

Servings: 4

Ingredients:
- ✓ 3 tomatoes, sliced
- ✓ 1 large avocado, sliced
- ✓ 8 kalamata olives

Directions:
- ❖ Arrange the tomato slices on a serving platter and place the avocado slices in the center.

Ingredients:
- ✓ ¼ lb buffalo mozzarella, sliced
- ✓ 2 tbsp pesto sauce
- ✓ 1 tbsp olive oil
- ❖ Arrange the olives around the avocado slices and drop mozzarella pieces onto the serving plate. Drizzle the pesto sauce and olive oil over everything and serve.

Nutrition: Calories 290, Fat: 25g, Net carbs: 4.3g, Protein: 9g

217)   Tuna salad with lettuce and olives

Preparation Time: 5 minutes

Servings: 2

Ingredients:
- ✓ 1 cup canned tuna, drained
- ✓ 1 tsp of onion flakes
- ✓ 3 tbsp mayonnaise

Directions:
- ❖ Combine tuna, mayonnaise and lime juice in a small bowl. Stir to combine. In a salad bowl, arrange shredded lettuce and onion flakes.

Ingredients:
- ✓ 1 cup romaine lettuce, shredded
- ✓ 1 tbsp lime juice
- ✓ 6 black olives, pitted and sliced
- ❖ Spread the tuna mixture over the top. Top with black olives and serve.

Nutrition: Calories 248, Fat: 20g, Net Carbs: 2g, Protein: 18.5g

218)   Cobb egg salad in lettuce cups

Preparation Time: 25 minutes

Servings: 4

Ingredients:

- ✓ 1 head of green lettuce, firm leaves removed for cups
- ✓ 2 chicken breasts, cut into pieces
- ✓ 1 tbsp olive oil
- ✓ Salt and black pepper to taste

Directions:

- ❖ Preheat oven to 400°F. Place chicken in a bowl, drizzle with olive oil and sprinkle with salt and black pepper. Cough to coat. Place the chicken on a baking sheet and spread it out evenly. Slide the baking sheet into the oven and bake the chicken until cooked through and golden brown for 8 minutes, stirring once.

Ingredients:

- ✓ 6 large eggs
- ✓ 2 tomatoes, seeded, chopped
- ✓ 6 tbsp Greek yogurt

- ❖ Boil the eggs in salted water for 10 minutes. Allow them to cool, peel and cut into pieces. Transfer to a salad bowl. Remove the chicken from the oven and add it to the salad bowl. Include the tomatoes and Greek yogurt and toss to combine. Layer 2 lettuce leaves each as cups and fill with 2 tbsp of egg salad each. Serve.

Nutrition: Calories 325, Fat 24.5g, Net Carbs 4g, Protein 21g

219)   Waffle sandwiches with gruyere and ham

Preparation Time: 20 minutes

Servings: 4

Ingredients:

- ✓ 4 slices smoked ham, chopped
- ✓ 4 tbsp butter, softened
- ✓ ½ cup Gruyere cheese, grated
- ✓ 6 eggs

Directions:

- ❖ In a bowl, mix the eggs, baking powder, thyme and butter. Place a waffle iron over medium heat, add ¼ cup of the batter and cook for 6 minutes until golden brown. Do the same with the remaining batter until you have 8 thin waffles.

Ingredients:

- ✓ ½ tsp baking powder
- ✓ ½ tsp dried thyme
- ✓ 4 slices tomato

- ❖ Lay a slice of tomato on one waffle, followed by a slice of ham, then top with ¼ of the grated cheese. Cover with another waffle, place the sandwich in the waffle iron and cook until the cheese melts. Repeat with remaining ingredients.

Nutrition: Calories 276; Net carbs 3.1g; Fat 22g; Protein 16g

220)   Baked chorizo with ricotta cheese

Preparation Time: 30 minutes

Servings: 6

Ingredients:

- ✓ 7 ounces Spanish chorizo, sliced
- ✓ 4 ounces ricotta cheese, crumbled

Directions:

- ❖ Preheat oven to 325 F. Spread chorizo on a wax paper-lined baking sheet and bake for 15 minutes until crispy

Ingredients:

- ✓ ¼ cup chopped parsley

- ❖ Remove from oven and allow to cool. Arrange on a serving platter. Add ricotta cheese and parsley.

Nutrition: Calories 172; Net carbohydrates: 0.2g; Fat: 13g; Protein: 5g

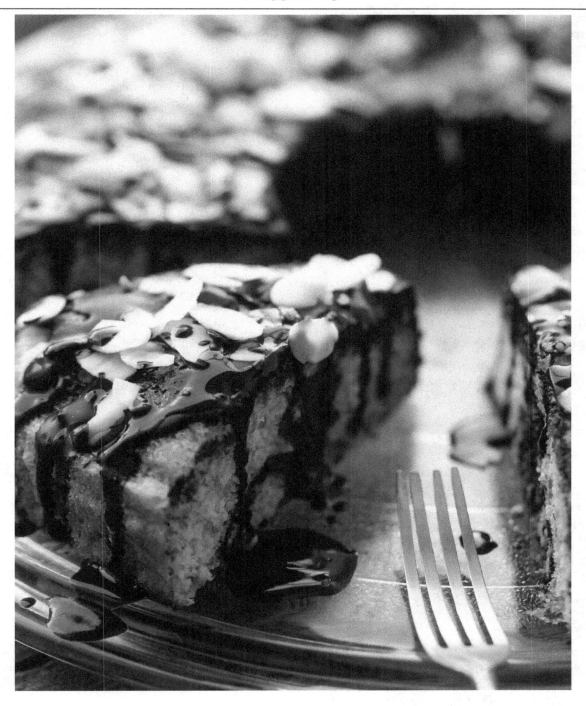

221) Coconut fat bombs

Preparation Time: 2 minutes + cooling time

Servings: 4

Ingredients:
- ✓ 2/3 cup coconut oil, melted
- ✓ 1 can of coconut milk (14 ounces)

Ingredients:
- ✓ 18 drops of liquid stevia
- ✓ 1 cup unsweetened coconut flakes
- ❖ Pour into silicone muffin molds and freeze for 1 hour to harden.

Directions:
- ❖ Mix the coconut oil with the milk and stevia. Stir in coconut flakes until well distributed.

Nutrition: Calories 214, fat 19g, net carbs 2g, protein 4g

222) Dark Chocolate Mochaccino Ice Bombs

Preparation Time: 5 minutes + cooling time

Servings: 4

Ingredients:
- ✓ ½ pound of cream cheese
- ✓ 4 tbsp powdered sweetener
- ✓ 2 ounces of strong coffee

Ingredients:
- ✓ 2 tbsp unsweetened cocoa powder
- ✓ 1 tbsp cocoa butter, melted
- ✓ 2 1/2 ounces melted dark chocolate
- ❖ . Mix in the melted cocoa butter and chocolate and coat the bombs with it. Freeze for 2 hours.

Directions:
- ❖ Combine the cream cheese, sweetener, coffee and cocoa powder in a food processor. Spread 2 tbsp of the mixture and place on a lined tray.

Nutrition: Calories Calories 127, Fat: 13g, Net Carbohydrates: 1.4g, Protein: 1.9g

223) Strawberry and ricotta parfait

Preparation Time: 10 minutes

Servings: 4

Ingredients:
- ✓ 2 cups strawberries, chopped
- ✓ 1 cup ricotta cheese

Ingredients:
- ✓ 2 tbsp sugar-free maple syrup
- ✓ 2 tbsp balsamic vinegar

Directions:
- ❖ Divide half of the strawberries among 4 small glasses and top with the ricotta.

- ❖ Drizzle with maple syrup, balsamic vinegar and finish with remaining strawberries. Serve.

Nutrition: Calories 164; Net carbs 3.1g; Fat 8.2g; Protein 7g

224) Creamy strawberry mousse

Preparation Time: 10 minutes + cooling time

Servings:

Ingredients:
- ✓ 2 cups frozen strawberries
- ✓ 2 tbsp sugar swerve

Ingredients:
- ✓ 1 large egg white
- ✓ 2 cups whipped cream
- ❖ Use an electric hand whisk to beat until the mixture is frothy. Pour mixture into dessert glasses and top with whipped cream and strawberries. Serve chilled.

Directions:
- ❖ Pour 1 ½ cups of strawberries into a blender and process until smooth. Add the swerve sugar and process further. Pour in the egg whites and transfer the mixture to a bowl.

Nutrition: Calories 145; Net carbohydrates 4.8g; Fat 6.8g; Protein 2g

225) Berry Clafoutis

Preparation Time: 45 minutes

Servings: 4

Ingredients:

- ✓ 4 eggs
- ✓ 2 tbsp coconut oil
- ✓ 2 cups berries
- ✓ 1 cup coconut milk

Ingredients:

- ✓ 1 cup almond flour
- ✓ ¼ cup sweetener
- ✓ ½ tsp vanilla powder
- ✓ 1 tbsp powdered sweetener
- ❖ Gently add the berries. Grease a flan pan with coconut oil and pour in the mixture. Bake for 35 minutes. Sprinkle with powdered sugar and serve.

Directions:

- ❖ Preheat oven to 350 F. Place all ingredients except coconut oil, berries and sweetener powder in a blender until smooth.

Nutrition: Calories 198; Net carbs 4.9g; Fat 16g; Protein 15g

226) Coconut and raspberry cheesecake

Preparation Time: 40 minutes + cooling time

Servings: 6

Ingredients:

- ✓ 2 egg whites
- ✓ 1 ¼ cups erythritol
- ✓ 3 cups desiccated coconut
- ✓ 1 tbsp coconut oil
- ✓ ¼ cup melted butter

Ingredients:

- ✓ 3 tbsp lemon juice
- ✓ 6 ounces raspberries
- ✓ 1 cup whipped cream
- ✓ 3 tbsp lemon juice
- ✓ 24 ounces of cream cheese
- ❖ Add lemon juice and remaining erythritol. In another bowl, beat the heavy cream with an electric mixer. Fold the whipped cream into the cream cheese mixture; stir in the raspberries. Spread the filling over the baked crust. Refrigerate for 4 hours. Serve.

Directions:

- ❖ Preheat oven to 350 F. Grease a baking sheet with coconut oil and line with baking paper. Mix egg whites, ¼ cup erythritol, coconut and butter until a crust forms and pour into the baking dish. Bake for 25 minutes. Allow to cool. Beat the cream cheese until smooth.

Nutrition: Calories 215; Net Carbs 3g; Fat 25g; Protein 5g

227) Peanut butter and chocolate ice cream bars

Preparation Time: approxi 4 hours and 20 minutes

Servings: 6

Ingredients:

- ✓ ¼ cup cocoa butter chunks, chopped
- ✓ 2 cups heavy whipping cream
- ✓ ⅔ cup peanut butter, softened
- ✓ 1 ½ cups almond milk

Ingredients:

- ✓ 1 tbsp vegetable glycerin
- ✓ 6 tbsp xylitol
- ✓ ¾ cup coconut oil
- ✓ 2 ounces unsweetened chocolate
- ❖ Mix coconut oil, cocoa butter, chocolate and remaining xylitol and microwave until melted; let cool slightly. Cut ice cream into bars. Dip into chocolate mixture. Serve.

Directions:

- ❖ Mix the heavy cream, peanut butter, almond milk, vegetable glycerin and half of the xylitol until smooth. Place in an ice cream maker and follow instructions. Spread the ice cream into a lined baking dish and freeze for 4 hours.

Nutrition: Calories 345 Net carbohydrates 5g; Fat 32g; Protein 4g

228) Lemon and yogurt mousse

Preparation Time: 5 minutes + cooling time

Servings:

Ingredients:

- ✓ 24 ounces plain yogurt, strained overnight in cheesecloth
- ✓ 2 cups powdered sugar swerve

Ingredients:

- ✓ 2 lemons, squeezed and peeled
- ✓ 1 cup whipped cream + extra for garnish

Directions:

- ❖ Whip plain yogurt in a bowl with a hand mixer until light and fluffy. Stir in the swerve sugar, lemon juice and salt. Add the whipped cream to combine.

- ❖ Pour mousse into serving cups and refrigerate for 1 hour. Swirl with more whipped cream and garnish with lemon zest.

Nutrition: Calories 223; Net Carbs 3g; Fat 18g; Protein 12g

229) Strawberry Chocolate Mousse

Preparation Time: 30 minutes

Servings: 4

Ingredients:

- ✓ 1 cup fresh strawberries, sliced
- ✓ 3 eggs
- ✓ 1 cup dark chocolate chips

Ingredients:

- ✓ 1 cup heavy cream
- ✓ 1 vanilla extract
- ✓ 1 tbsp sugar swerve

Directions:

- ❖ Melt chocolate in a microwave-safe bowl in the microwave for 1 minute; let cool for 8 minutes. In a bowl, whip heavy cream until very smooth.

- ❖ Whisk in the eggs, vanilla extract and sugar swerve. Add the cooled chocolate. Divide the mousse between glasses, top with the strawberry and chill in the refrigerator. Serve.

Nutrition: Calories 400; Net Carbs 1.7g; Fat 25g; Protein 8g

230) Maple Lemon Cake

Preparation Time: 30 minutes

Servings:

Ingredients:

- ✓ 4 eggs
- ✓ 1 cup sour cream
- ✓ 2 lemons, peeled and squeezed
- ✓ 1 tsp vanilla extract
- ✓ 2 cups almond flour
- ✓ 2 tbsp coconut flour

Ingredients:

- ✓ 2 tbsp baking powder
- ✓ ½ cup xylitol
- ✓ 1 tsp cardamom powder
- ✓ ½ tsp ground ginger
- ✓ A pinch of salt
- ✓ ¼ cup maple syrup

Directions:

- ❖ Preheat oven to 400 F. Grease a cake pan with melted butter. In a bowl, beat the eggs, sour cream, lemon juice and vanilla extract until smooth. In another bowl, whisk together the almond and coconut flours, baking powder, xylitol, cardamom, ginger, salt, lemon zest and half of the maple syrup.

- ❖ Combine both mixtures until smooth and pour the batter into the baking dish. Bake for 25 minutes or until a toothpick inserted comes out clean. Transfer to a wire rack, let cool and drizzle with remaining maple syrup. Serve in slices.

Nutrition: Calories 441; Net Carbs 8.5g; Fat 29g; Protein 33g

231) Flan with whipped cream

Preparation Time: 10 minutes + cooling time

Servings: 4

Ingredients:
- ✓ ⅓ cup erythritol, for the caramel
- ✓ 2 cups almond milk
- ✓ 4 eggs
- ✓ 1 tbsp vanilla

Ingredients:
- ✓ 1 tbsp lemon zest
- ✓ ½ cup erythritol, for the custard
- ✓ 2 cups heavy whipping cream
- ✓ Mint leaves, for serving
- ❖ Pour enough hot water into the baking dish to halfway up the sides of the cups. Bake at 345 F for 45 minutes. Remove the ramekins and place them in the refrigerator for 4 hours. Take a knife and run slowly around the edges to spill onto plates. Serve with spoonfuls of cream and mint leaves.

Directions:
- ❖ Heat the erythritol for the caramel in a pan. Add 2-3 tbsp of water and bring to a boil. Reduce heat and cook until caramel turns golden brown. Carefully divide among 4 metal cups. Allow them to cool. In a bowl, mix the eggs, remaining erythritol, lemon zest and vanilla. Add the almond milk and beat again until combined. Pour the cream into the caramel lined cups and place in a baking dish.

Nutrition: Calories 169; Net carbs 1.7g; Fat 10g; Protein 7g

232) Chocolate and walnut cookies

Preparation Time: 30 minutes

Servings: 4

Ingredients:
- ✓ 2/3 cup dark chocolate chips
- ✓ 4 ounces butter, softened
- ✓ 2 tbsp swerve sugar
- ✓ 2 tbsp brown sugar swerve
- ✓ 1 egg

Ingredients:
- ✓ 1 tsp vanilla extract
- ✓ ½ cup almond flour
- ✓ ½ tsp baking soda
- ✓ ½ cup chopped walnuts

Directions:
- ❖ Preheat oven to 350 F. In a bowl, beat butter, swerve sugar and swerve brown sugar until smooth. Beat in the egg and stir in the vanilla extract. In another bowl, combine the almond flour with the baking soda and mix into the wet ingredients. Add the chocolate chips and walnuts.

- ❖ Spoon full tbsp of batter onto a greased baking sheet, leaving 2 inches of space between each spoonful. Press each batter to flatten slightly. Bake for 15 minutes. Transfer to a rack to cool completely. Serve.

Nutrition: Calories 430; Net carbohydrates 3.5g; Fat 42g; Protein 6g

233) Quick Blueberry Sorbet

Preparation Time: 15 minutes + cooling time

Servings: 4

Ingredients:
- ✓ 4 cups frozen blueberries
- ✓ 1 cup sugar swerve

Ingredients:
- ✓ ½ lemon, squeezed
- ✓ ½ tsp salt
- ❖ Chill for 3 hours. Pour cooled juice into an ice cream maker and strain until mixture resembles ice cream. Spoon into a bowl and chill further for 3 hours.

Directions:
- ❖ In a blender, add blueberries, swerve, lemon juice and salt; process until smooth. Strain through a strainer into a bowl.

Nutrition: Calories 178; Net Carbs 2.3g; Fat 1g; Protein 0.6g

234)   Trifle of mixed berries

Preparation Time: 3 minutes + cooling time

Servings: 4

Ingredients:

- ✓ ½ cup walnuts, toasted
- ✓ 1 avocado, chopped
- ✓ 1 cup mascarpone cheese, softened

Directions:

- ❖ In four dessert glasses, divide half of the mascarpone, half of the berries (mixed), half of the walnuts and half of the avocado.

Ingredients:

- ✓ 1 cup fresh blueberries
- ✓ 1 cup fresh raspberries
- ✓ 1 cup fresh blackberries
- ❖ Repeat the layering process a second time to finish the ingredients. Cover the glasses with plastic wrap and refrigerate for 45 minutes until fairly firm.

Nutrition: Calories 321, Fat 28.5g, Net Carbohydrates 8.3g, Protein 9.8g

235)   Creamy Coconut Kiwi Drink

Preparation Time: 3 minutes

Servings: 4

Ingredients:

- ✓ 5 kiwis, picked pulp
- ✓ 2 tbsp of erythritol
- ✓ 2 cups unsweetened coconut milk

Directions:

- ❖ In a blender, process the kiwis, erythritol, milk, cream and ice cubes until smooth, about 3 minutes.

Ingredients:

- ✓ 2 cups of coconut cream
- ✓ 7 ice cubes
- ✓ Mint leaves for garnish
- ❖ Pour into four serving glasses, garnish with mint leaves and serve.

Nutrition: Calories 351, Fat 28g, Net Carbs 9.7g, Protein 16g

236)   Walnut Cookies

Preparation Time: 15 minutes

Servings: 12

Ingredients:

- ✓ 1 egg
- ✓ 2 cups ground pecans
- ✓ ¼ cup sweetener

Directions:

- ❖ Preheat oven to 350°F. Mix ingredients, except walnuts, until combined. Make 20 balls with the dough and press them with your thumb onto a lined cookie sheet.

Ingredients:

- ✓ ½ tsp baking soda
- ✓ 1 tbsp butter
- ✓ 20 walnut halves
- ❖ Top each cookie with a walnut half. Bake for about 12 minutes.

Nutrition: Calories 101, Fat: 11g, Net Carbs: 0.6g, Protein: 1.6g

237)   Chocolate Bark with Almonds

Preparation Time: 5 minutes + cooling time

Servings: 12

Ingredients:

- ✓ ½ cup toasted almonds, chopped
- ✓ ½ cup butter
- ✓ 10 drops of stevia

Directions:

- ❖ Melt the butter and chocolate together, in the microwave, for 90 seconds. Remove and stir in the stevia. Line a cookie sheet with wax paper and spread the chocolate evenly.

Ingredients:

- ✓ ¼ tsp salt
- ✓ ½ cup unsweetened coconut flakes
- ✓ 4 ounces dark chocolate
- ❖ Scatter the almonds on top, coconut flakes and sprinkle with salt. Place in the refrigerator for 1 hour.

Nutrition: Calories 161, Fat: 15.3g, Net Carbohydrates: 1.9g, Protein: 1.9g

238)   Raspberry Sorbet

Preparation Time: 10 minutes + cooling time

Servings: 1

Ingredients:

- ✓ ¼ tsp vanilla extract
- ✓ 1 package of gelatin, unsweetened
- ✓ 1 tbsp heavy whipping cream

Directions:

- ❖ Cover gelatin with cold water in a small bowl. Allow to dissolve for 5 minutes. Transfer to a blender.

Ingredients:

- ✓ 2 tbsp raspberry puree
- ✓ 1 ½ cups crushed ice

- ❖ Add remaining ingredients and ⅓ cup cold water. Blend until smooth and freeze for at least 2 hours.

Nutrition: Calories 173, Fat: 10g, Net Carbohydrates: 3.7g, Protein: 4g

239)   Wonderful berry pudding

Preparation Time: 45 minutes

Servings: 2

Ingredients:

- ✓ 1 cup almond flour
- ✓ 2 tbsp of lemon juice
- ✓ 2 cups blueberries
- ✓ 2 tbsp baking powder
- ✓ ½ tsp ground nutmeg
- ✓ ½ cup coconut milk
- ✓ 3 tbsp stevia

Directions:

- ❖ In a greased heatproof dish, mix blueberries and lemon juice, stir a little and spread over the bottom.
- ❖ In a bowl, mix flour with nutmeg, stevia, baking powder, vanilla, ghee, flaxseed meal, arrowroot and milk, mix well again and spread over blueberries.

Ingredients:

- ✓ 1 tbsp flax meal mixed with 1 tbsp water
- ✓ 3 tbsp melted ghee
- ✓ 1 tbsp vanilla extract
- ✓ 1 tbsp arrowroot powder
- ✓ 1 cup cold water

- ❖ Put the water in the Instant Pot, add the trivet and heatproof dish, cover and cook on high heat for 35 minutes.
- ❖ Let pudding cool, transfer to dessert bowls and serve.

Nutrition: Calories 220 | Fat: 4g | Carbohydrates: 9g | Protein: 6g | Fiber: 4g | Sugar: 2g

240)   Orange Dessert

Preparation Time: 45 minutes

Servings: 2

Ingredients:

- ✓   1 ¾ cups water
- ✓   1 tsp baking powder
- ✓   1 cup coconut flour
- ✓   2 tbsp stevia
- ✓   ½ tbsp cinnamon powder
- ✓   3 tbsp coconut oil, melted

Ingredients:

- ✓   ½ cup coconut milk
- ✓   ½ cup pecans, chopped
- ✓   ½ cup raisins
- ✓   ½ cup orange peel, grated
- ✓   ¾ cup orange juice

Directions:

- ❖   In a bowl, mix flour with stevia, baking powder, cinnamon, 2 tbsp oil, milk, pecans and raisins; stir and transfer to a greased heatproof dish.
- ❖   Heat a small skillet over medium-high heat, mix ¾ cup water with the orange juice, orange zest and the rest of the oil, stir, bring to a boil and pour over the pecan mixture.

- ❖   Place 1 cup of water in the Instant Pot, add the heatproof dish, cover and cook on High for 30 minutes.
- ❖   Serve cold.

Nutrition: Calories 142 | Fat: 3g | Carbohydrates: 3g | Protein: 3g | Fiber: 1g | Sugar: 1g

241)   Great Pumpkin Dessert

Preparation Time: 40 minutes

Servings: 2

Ingredients:

- ✓   1 and ½ tsp baking powder
- ✓   2 cups of coconut flour
- ✓   ½ tsp baking soda
- ✓   ¼ tsp ground nutmeg
- ✓   1 tsp cinnamon powder
- ✓   ¼ tsp ginger, grated
- ✓   1 cup water

Ingredients:

- ✓   1 tbsp coconut oil, melted
- ✓   1 egg white
- ✓   1 tbsp vanilla extract
- ✓   1 cup pumpkin puree
- ✓   2 tbsp stevia
- ✓   1 tbsp lemon juice

Directions:

- ❖   In a bowl, flour with baking powder, baking soda, cinnamon, ginger, nutmeg, oil, egg white, ghee, vanilla extract, pumpkin puree, stevia and lemon juice, mix well and transfer this to a greased cake pan.

- ❖   Put the water in the Instant Pot, add the trivet, add the cake pan, cover and bake on High for 30 minutes.
- ❖   Allow cake to cool, cut and serve.

Nutrition: Calories 180 | Fat: 3g | Carbohydrates: 3g | Protein: 4g | Fiber: 2g | Sugar: 0g

242) Merry Berry

Preparation Time: 6 minutes

Servings: 4

Ingredients:

- ✓ 1 cup strawberries + extra for garnish
- ✓ 1 ½ cups blackberries
- ✓ 1 cup blueberries

Directions:

- ❖ For extra strawberries for garnish, make a single deep cut on their sides; set aside. Add blackberries, strawberries, blueberries, beets and ice cubes to smoothie maker.

Ingredients:

- ✓ 2 small beets, peeled and chopped
- ✓ 2/3 cup ice cubes
- ✓ 1 lime, squeezed
- ❖ Blend ingredients on high speed until smooth and frothy, about 60 seconds. Add the lime juice and blend for 30 seconds more. Pour the drink into tall smoothie glasses, secure the reserved strawberries on the rim of each glass, stick a straw in and serve the drink immediately.

Nutrition: Calories 83, Fat 3g, Net Carbs 8g, Protein 2.7g

243) Cinnamon Cookies

Preparation Time: 25 minutes

Servings: 4

Ingredients:

- ✓ Cookies
- ✓ 2 cups almond flour
- ✓ ½ tsp baking soda
- ✓ ¾ cup sweetener
- ✓ ½ cup butter, softened

Directions:

- ❖ Preheat oven to 350°F. Combine all cookie ingredients in a bowl. Make 16 balls with the dough and flatten them with your hands. Combine the cinnamon and erythritol.

Ingredients:

- ✓ A pinch of salt
- ✓ Coating
- ✓ 2 tbsp erythritol sweetener
- ✓ 1 tsp cinnamon

- ❖ Dip the cookies into the cinnamon mixture and place them on a lined baking sheet. Bake for 15 minutes, until crispy.

Nutrition: Calories 134, Fat: 13g, Net Carbs: 1.5g, Protein: 3g

244) Vanilla Frappuccino

Preparation Time: 6 minutes

Servings: 4

Ingredients:

- ✓ 3 cups unsweetened vanilla almond milk, chilled Unsweetened chocolate chips for garnish
- ✓ 2 tbsp sugar swerve
- ✓ 1 ½ cups heavy cream, chilled

Directions:

- ❖ Combine almond milk, swerve sugar, heavy cream, vanilla bean and xanthan gum in blender and process on high speed for 1 minute until smooth.

Ingredients:

- ✓ 1 vanilla bean
- ✓ ¼ tsp xanthan gum

- ❖ Pour into tall shake glasses, sprinkle with chocolate chips and serve immediately.

Nutrition: Calories 193, Fat 14g, Net Carbs 6g, Protein 15g

245) Peanut Butter Pecan Ice Cream

Preparation Time: 36 minutes + cooling time

Servings: 4

Ingredients:

- ✓ ½ cup swerve confectioners sweetener
- ✓ 2 cups heavy cream
- ✓ 1 tbsp of erythritol
- ✓ ½ cup plain peanut butter

Ingredients:

- ✓ 1 tbsp olive oil
- ✓ 2 egg yolks
- ✓ ½ cup pecans, chopped

Directions:

- ❖ Heat the heavy cream with the peanut butter, olive oil and erythritol in a small skillet over low heat without boiling for about 3 minutes. Remove from heat. In a bowl, beat egg yolks until creamy.

- ❖ Stir the eggs into the cream mixture. Continue stirring until a thick batter has formed, about 3 minutes. Pour the cream mixture into a bowl. Place in the refrigerator for 30 minutes. Stir in confectioners' sweetener.
- ❖ Pour mixture into ice cream maker and churn according to manufacturer's instructions. Stir in pecan later and spoon mixture into baking dish. Freeze for 2 hours before serving.

Nutrition: Calories 302, Fat 32g, Net Carbs 2g, Protein 5g

246) Coffee Fat Bombs

Preparation Time: 3 minutes + cooling time

Servings: 6

Ingredients:

- ✓ 6 tbsp prepared coffee at room temperature
- ✓ 1 ½ cups mascarpone cheese
- ✓ ½ cup melted butter

Ingredients:

- ✓ 3 tbsp unsweetened cocoa powder
- ✓ ¼ cup erythritol

Directions:

- ❖ Beat mascarpone, butter, cocoa powder, erythritol and coffee with a hand mixer until creamy and fluffy, about 1 minute.

- ❖ Fill muffin pans and freeze for 3 hours until firm.

Nutrition: Calories 145, fat 14g, net carbs 2g, protein 4g

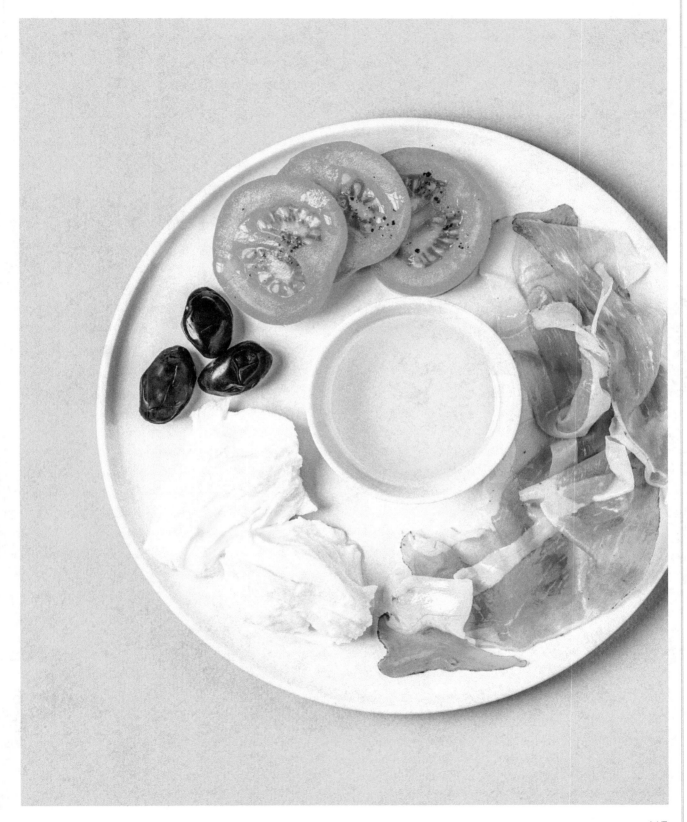

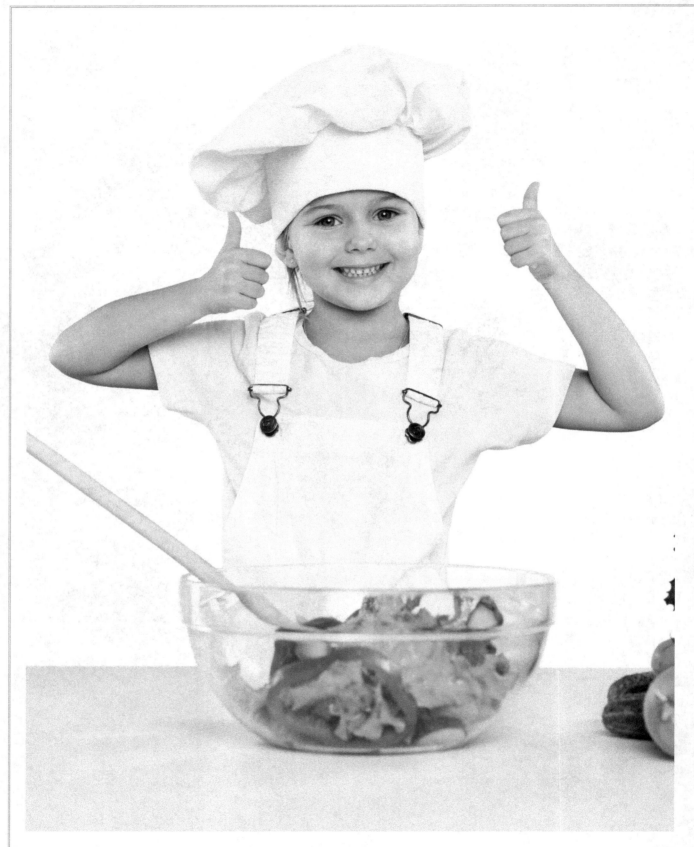

AUTHOR BIBLIOGRAPHY

THE PALEO DIET FOR MEN: The Guide with 150+ Grain- and Gluten-Free Recipes to Lose Weight and Start Whole-Foods Lifestyle!

THE PALEO DIET FOR WOMEN: 120+ Recipes to Discover the Secrets of Rapid Weight Loss and A Healthy Lifestyle Using the Paleo Diet!

THE PALEO DIET COOKBOOK: 120+ Tasty and Wholesome Recipes that Combine Paleo and Vegan Diet to Eating Well, Lose Weight, and Feeling Vibrant!

THE PALEO DIET FOR KIDS: 120+ Ultimate Paleo Recipes All Kid-Friendly to Become a Superheroes! All Paleo and Healthy -Based Food!

THE PALEO DIET FOR BEGINNERS: The Unique Guide to The Paleo Diet: 120+ Easy Recipes to Make Paleo Cooking Easy! regain your energy today!

THE PALEO DIET FOR COUPLE: 2 Books in 1: THE SECRETS OF RAPID WEIGHT LOSS AND A HEALTHY LIFESTYLE USING THE PALEO DIET! 200+ Wholesome, Easy to Follow and Delicious Recipes!

THE PALEO DIET FOR STUDENTS: 2 Books in 1: PALEO Diet GUIDE for Beginners: An easy guide to the with over 200 Delicious Quick and Easy Recipes.

THE PALEO DIET BASICS: 2 Books in 1: The Guide for Beginners to Lose Weight Quickly and Regain Confidence, Cut Cholesterol, and Feel Young Again! Improve your Health Easily! 200+ FANTASTIC RECIPES TO TRY!

THE PALEO FOR ATHLETE: The 200+ Simplest High-Protein and Low-Carb Paleo Recipes to start Fitness and Tone your Body to The Top!

CONCLUSIONS

The Paleo diet is a lifestyle answer that is steadily gaining popularity these days. Many people are finding this diet very beneficial to their health. It is a natural diet that focuses on whole and unprocessed foods.

With the Paleo diet, you can lose weight and feel healthier. The Paleo diet is low in sugar. It is free of grains, dairy, legumes, refined carbohydrates, and processed foods. This means you will eat natural foods rich in vitamins, minerals, antioxidants, and fiber.

The Paleo diet helps in the prevention of various diseases. Some benefits of the Paleo diet include an improved immune system and a reduced chance of developing cancer and heart disease. The Paleo diet is a way of eating that became popular in the early 2000s. It is a lifestyle that hunter-gatherers practiced for millions of years before agriculture. One of the key ideas is that we have evolved to eat foods that are in season. It's a way to ensure we get nutrients from our food. A simple way to implement this way of eating is to find whole, fresh foods in season. The Paleo diet does not encourage processed foods, fast foods, or refined sugars or oils. It is considered ideal for keeping the mind and body healthy. It encourages the consumption of fresh foods and minimizes exposure to chemicals such as preservatives and artificial additives. The Paleo diet is a way of life for Paleolithic humans. This means that the way they ate differed from the way we eat today. This diet is designed to mimic the eating habits of our ancestors. The Paleo diet focuses on eating foods that are rich in vitamins and minerals. These foods include fish, meat, vegetables, fruits, nuts, and seeds. This diet also encourages low glycaemic index fruits and vegetables.

As beneficial as this diet can be to your health, it also has drawbacks. For example, individuals who follow the Paleo diet may suffer from nutrient deficiencies. This type of diet can also lead to a higher incidence of health problems such as acne and cancer.

However, you address these issues, you need to know what the Paleo diet is and how it is used today.